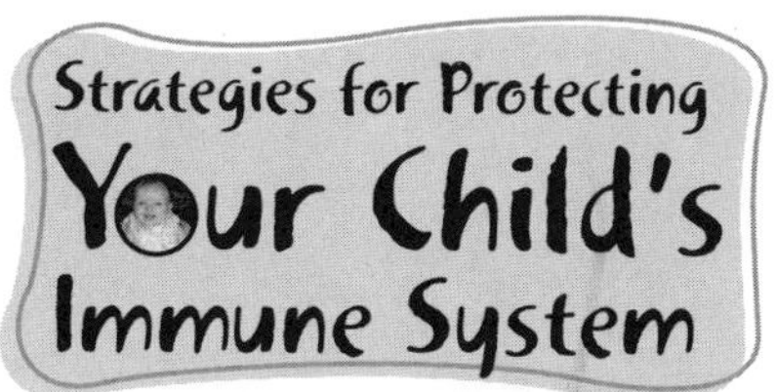

Tools for Parents and Parents-To-Be

NORTH SHORE PUBLIC LIBRARY
3 0651 00240 9161

Strategies for Protecting Your Child's Immune System

Tools for Parents and Parents-To-Be

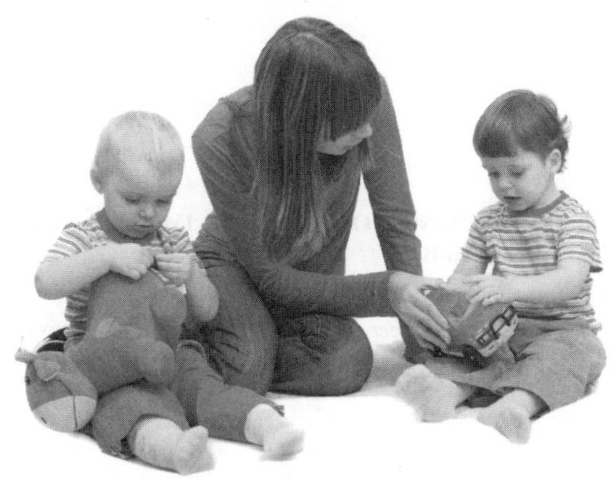

Rodney R Dietert
Cornell University, USA

Janice Dietert
Performance Plus Consulting, USA

NORTH SHORE PUBLIC LIBRARY
250 ROUTE 25 A
SHOREHAM, NEW YORK 11786 - 2190

World Scientific

NEW JERSEY • LONDON • SINGAPORE • BEIJING • SHANGHAI • HONG KONG • TAIPEI • CHENNAI

Published by

World Scientific Publishing Co. Pte. Ltd.
5 Toh Tuck Link, Singapore 596224
USA office: 27 Warren Street, Suite 401-402, Hackensack, NJ 07601
UK office: 57 Shelton Street, Covent Garden, London WC2H 9HE

British Library Cataloguing-in-Publication Data
A catalogue record for this book is available from the British Library.

STRATEGIES FOR PROTECTING YOUR CHILD'S IMMUNE SYSTEM
Tools for Parents and Parents-To-Be

Copyright © 2010 by World Scientific Publishing Co. Pte. Ltd.
All rights reserved. This book, or parts thereof, may not be reproduced in any form or by any means, electronic or mechanical, including photocopying, recording or any information storage and retrieval system now known or to be invented, without written permission from the Publisher.

For photocopying of material in this volume, please pay a copying fee through the Copyright Clearance Center, Inc., 222 Rosewood Drive, Danvers, MA 01923, USA. In this case permission to photocopy is not required from the publisher.

ISBN-13 978-981-4287-09-8 (pbk)
ISBN-10 981-4287-09-1 (pbk)

Typeset by Stallion Press
Email: enquiries@stallionpress.com

Printed in Singapore by World Scientific Printers

To our children Michele Melligan, Grant Dietert and Matthew Dietert and to any children they have or may have

Contents

Acknowledgments

We thank the following individuals for their helpful suggestions while preparing this book:

Arlene Alderman
Dr. Randall Corey
Bethanie Dietert
Beverly Dietert
David Kessler
Dr. Stephen Penningroth
John Richmond
Harold Salter

Photos used by permission of Bethanie Dietert, Grant Dietert, Ralph Dietert, and Joy Quek.

Introduction

This book is not about medical advice or medical decisions. Those are strictly between you, the reader, and your physician. This book is about reducing health risks for your child's immune system, and it provides strategies you can use based on the latest scientific research. The information on immune risk provided in this book is our effort to give readers a science-based equivalent of a consumer's report for helping your baby develop a well-balanced immune system.

The truth is that most people don't give much thought to the immune system. The average person understands that when they have an infection or the flu, their immune system is what fights it off and helps them get better. Because of HIV/AIDS, we've all seen what happens when the immune system is severely compromised. But when pollen fills the air and your hayfever acts up, is your immune system the first thing on your mind? How about when you can't get a breath of air, and you reach for your inhaler? Perhaps these common ailments prompt some thought of the immune system. What about when the body turns against itself, as in the case of lupus or type I diabetes? Those illnesses often set off serious concern about immune issues, yet they don't help create better understanding of how the diseases develop. Least understood from the viewpoint of the immune system are conditions like childhood leukemia, multiple sclerosis, chronic fatigue syndrome, sarcoidosis, Parkinson's disease, autism and autism spectrum disorders (ASDs), atherosclerosis and male infertility. Is it really possible for all of these conditions to have an immune component?

If all of the research from the past five to ten years is accurate, the picture that has formed answers that question with a resounding, yes. Not only is the immune system intimately involved in the development of many illnesses, but research has shown that this involvement occurs far earlier than has ever been suspected. A tremendous wealth of data has begun to show that while the baby is still in its mother's womb, at the very period in time when the immune system is developing (across all trimesters), the immune system is the most vulnerable to often permanent, potentially irreversible damage that will affect the child for life.

Why has it taken so long to discover this unsettling reality? The reason is that knowledge about damage to the immune system is relatively new. When the first observations were reported 30 to 35 years ago, the pioneers in the field did the best they could given the level of understanding and technology at that time. They knew that exposure to a toxin during the first three months of pregnancy could completely suppress the immune system and kill the fetus. In fact, up until just a few years ago regulators looked at profound immunosuppression as the principle cause for concern when examining the possible impact chemicals or pharmaceuticals could have on the immune system. Until recently, death due to infection or cancer was the main negative outcome tied to immune system trauma.

However, over the last five years, greatly improved research techniques and technologies have allowed researchers to understand just how intricate, interwoven and finely tuned the immune system really is. We now know: 1) what comprises the immune system, 2) the many different ways it can be damaged, 3) when it begins to develop and 4) many of the developmental stages it goes through while the baby is in utero. Some of these stages will never be duplicated again in the individual's lifetime. Now we're able to see changes that affect the developing immune system yet don't kill the fetus and to track the outcome of these changes over a lifetime. We're beginning to discover how permanent changes in the developing immune system combine with genetic predisposition for illness to create chronic lifelong health challenges. We are learning that there is no safe period during pregnancy to smoke, drink alcohol, be exposed to unsafe levels of pesticides or even to take some medications and herbs.

All too slowly, researchers have developed the wherewithal to detect the harm, track the changes, and witness the breakdown in health or cognitive functions as the child grows older. With this new understanding comes the recognition that the impact of toxic exposures during pregnancy can be compounded over a lifetime. Enter the era of Developmental Immunotoxicology, the era when researchers now understand that certain environmental exposures of the fetus in utero may make it impossible for the child's immune system to mature sufficiently to protect it from the normal immune challenges he/she will face throughout life. Instead, its immune system will often remain frozen in an almost fetal state, acting like a pre-born fetus' immune system in an adult body as it responds to real-world viruses and bacteria. Sometimes it will fight off intruders, but just as likely it will fight against itself. Often, it resides in a highly revved up state as if it's always under attack when no attacker is present, and this creates chronic inflammation throughout the body. Yet, when the individual is exposed to a real virus or bacteria, rather than going into an even higher gear to fight off infection, the immune system shuts down instead, much like your computer when you have opened one too many websites at once. It reacts in entirely unpredictable ways to vaccinations and immunizations causing harm in various parts of the body and to different systems. Sometimes coming in contact again with the toxin that created the damage before birth will cause an unpredictable response. An immune system that was hit by a toxic exposure in the womb is an immune system gone haywire later in life.

Let's take the case of JM as an example. Her mother worked as a proofreader in a publishing company in the 1950's and 60's. In those days, inks were made with heavy metals like lead, mercury, chromium and hexavalent cadmium. Nasty stuff for mom; even nastier for a baby. The proofing room was upstairs from the printing presses, and ventilation in those days carried fumes upward. Plus, mom received wet copy to proof immediately, and a quick return was in order to get the manuscript back to the typesetters so the book could be printed. She was pregnant for several months before finally taking maternity leave.

The pregnancy itself was uneventful and a small daughter was born. Within days, however, problems began to arise. First, an allergy to cow's milk created intense colic for the first six months until solid foods were introduced. And the child never seemed able to fight off infections. Not only did they come rolling in, colds, flus, strep throat, bronchitis, but many required repeated rounds of increasingly stronger antibiotics.

As the child grew, her health problems did not improve. In fact, her parents and her doctor had to start being very careful about which vaccinations and medications she received. When she was just three or four years old, she had an intense, adverse reaction to the MMR vaccine and came close to being hospitalized. She never did get a tetanus shot, even into adulthood because nobody felt "lucky" enough on any given day that she would react reasonably to it.

JM continued the pattern of "sickliness" as she went through school. She didn't just get double mumps (in spite of having been vaccinated against it) and chicken pox; she got them one right after another in quick succession. Not a year went by without chronic bronchitis all winter. The continuous use of antibiotics taken repeatedly took a toll, and she was hospitalized near death when only eight because she could no longer keep food or drink down, her gut bacteria had been so destroyed.

Even in her teens and 20s, JM continued to develop new and unusual patterns of illness. Her milk allergy had been mild but by her mid-20s, it was joined by an allergy to beef so severe that even tiny amounts elicited a strong reaction. She was hyper-sensitive to many medications, and her doctors had to be increasingly careful about what they prescribed for her. To her list of year-round allergies she added an allergy to tobacco smoke that nearly made her pass out at the scent of stale smoke on clothing.

She had developed mild fibromyalgia in high school that gradually worsened. By her late 20s, she had irritable bowel syndrome. Twenty years later she would add chronic fatigue syndrome to the list of continuing challenges, and the fibromyalgia worsened to the point that it was now a force to be reckoned with. All of her ailments had a component of uncontrollable inflammation that contributed to bouts of clinical depression and chronic insomnia.

Because of her childhood susceptibility to the strep bacteria and chronic sinus infections, she had become resistant to all but two of the strongest antibiotics. It had been a life of chronic rolling infections and increasingly more devastating illnesses, most of them focused on one immune challenge after another, challenges it seemed her immune system was not capable of handling appropriately.

This, by the way, is a real case history, though no names will be revealed. While the large number of illnesses may seem unusual and the development of an illness after receiving vaccination against it contradictory, such interrelated health problems are more common than we think (see Chapters 11 and 19).

Part I — The Basic Science

Chapter 1 — Toxicology 101

Introduction

The whole purpose of this book is to provide information that can help readers discern what factors in the environment are likely to promote effective immunity and corresponding good health in their children from those that are likely to contribute to immune problems and chronic disease. Individual variation certainly exists, and one's genetic background can influence metabolism, organ sensitivity and the impact of chemical exposures and dietary intake. But there is also information that is generally applicable to all pregnant women and children and can help in creating a safer environment for the child's developing immune system. One important step in this process is the identification of what is harmful and what is not, also known as toxicology.

For our purpose of discussing human health risk and particularly that of our children, toxicology can be defined as the study of the adverse health effects resulting from exposure to chemical, physical or biological agents. The interaction between the body and the external environment includes a variety of encounters with chemical, physical and biological factors ranging from pesticides and solvents to drugs and toxin-containing infectious agents. These interactions occur through the foods we eat, the air we breathe, the water we drink and the surroundings we and others create.

These surroundings can range from those found in our home (clothing, cleaning agents, toys and furniture) to those in our workplace environment (computers, copiers, air handling systems, machinery) and those in our neighborhoods (daycare centers, traffic, roadways, shopping areas, golf courses, farms, parks and skyscrapers). Everything we encounter, whether through our lungs, on our skin, via our mouth or through our eyes, becomes an environmental exposure worthy of examination. But each element is not necessarily of equal concern. Some elements carry a significant risk that they may harm the immune system. Other exposures have very little risk for immune damage. Some exposures are beneficial and even necessary for good health. Making those distinctions is why toxicology developed as a science. This concept of risk is discussed further in the next chapter.

The interactions between the body and environmental factors generally follow very simple rules. Some exposures are useful and may play a critical role in promoting good health. Others are problematic and can damage the health of our children. Some exposures are not only beneficial but are necessary for survival (e.g., intake of certain vitamins and minerals). The body, including its immune system, needs certain dietary building blocks or it cannot survive. For example, we must have protein for our immune cells to continue to function and maintain healthy muscles.

At the other extreme, a number of exposures are likely to be harmful for virtually everyone regardless of age, gender or genetic background (e.g., exposure to cyanide or sarin gas). However, there is also a middle ground. There are some environmental factors that can be dangerous, but only for some groups of people. For example, exposure to cytomegalovirus is usually not a big problem for people with a healthy immune system. But for the very young, the very elderly and those with weakened immune systems (e.g., AIDS or chemotherapy patients), exposure to that virus can be life threatening. There are also some substances that may be very toxic but not every exposure to them presents an equal danger. An example of this is botulism toxin.

Botulism toxin is produced by the bacterium, *Clostridium botulinum.* It is also one of the most potent toxins known. Why were people in older generations taught never to buy a canned good with the sides bulging out? Because the bulges were a result of a broken or improper seal and presented the risk of botulism contamination. In the past, people were taught that these products should be avoided at all costs. Or should they?

Ironically, nowadays some people actually pay good money to be exposed to one of the most dangerous toxins we know. The exposures come in the form of BOTOX treatments. Miniscule amounts of the botulism toxin are injected into small areas of the body (generally the face) for cosmetic and medical purposes. The botulism toxin stops signals between the nerves and muscles. This can be used to treat medical problems such as Bell's palsy, lazy eye or cerebral palsy. Of course it has also been used cosmetically to remove wrinkles. But the trick is to ensure the toxic action is only in the local nerves and muscle and can never reach the brain.

Another extremely deadly toxin has also been used for medical treatments. Ricin toxin is the product of castor beans and is a public health concern since it has been produced by terrorist organizations seeking to chemically attack and destroy large populations. But the toxin has medical applications when it can be delivered to cells we want to kill. Very small amounts of the ricin toxin are used to target cancer cells in cancer therapy. Antibodies can be used to direct the ricin poison directly to the cancer cells. In spite of the positive uses for both botulism toxin and ricin toxin, there still remain significant dangers if we encounter them outside of these highly specialized circumstances.

So the trick in toxicology is to know which environmental exposures fall into high health risk categories. What needs to be considered to make this determination? Here are some of the questions that get asked along the way.

1) What is the nature of the environmental factor?
2) What is the way in which the body handles or processes it?
3) How much time does it or its by-products spend in the body?
4) What reactions does this factor undergo in the body?

These questions and the resulting answers help us to place an environmental factor into different categories of potential danger.

One of the misconceptions about chemicals is that we can easily divide them all into a world of inherently good chemicals or despicably evil chemicals. For a few selected chemicals with historic industrial benefits (e.g., the heavy metals lead, mercury, cadmium, arsenic and the dioxins), it is challenging to find any beneficial, let alone "safe" levels.

But for the vast majority of chemicals, blanket good vs. evil labels simply don't apply. The reality is that for most chemicals and drugs, significant health risks occur only for some levels of exposure while other exposure levels are either safe (innocuous to our health) or may be beneficial if not required for good health (e.g., iron, zinc, and vitamin D). In these cases, there is no good or evil label that is useful, only good or bad doses of exposure. For example, one might think that in terms of health, oxygen is inherently good, mercury is inherently evil. But there is more to this story. It is the dose that makes the poison.

The Dose Makes the Poison

In 16th century Germany, a physician and alchemist first began to detail the impact of minerals on human health. This doctor, who revolutionized Medieval thinking about environment and health, eventually became known simply as Paracelsus. Paracelsus recognized that the intake of some minerals was required for good health while other mineral exposures produced illness and even death. He also noted that only certain levels of mineral intake were effective for promoting improved health. Paracelsus essentially became an early version of what we would now call a compounding pharmacist. Among his most significant accomplishments was the coining of what in English translation has become the motto of modern toxicology "the dose makes the poison." This is the entire basis of the field of toxicology, which is founded on the concepts established by Paracelsus. We understand that chemicals and drugs can be safe at some levels of exposure and dangerous at others. Of importance is learning what safe doses are, what dangerous doses are and when we might encounter each of them.

Too Much of a Good Thing

Oxygen is essential for human life; everyone agrees with this. Our atmosphere contains approximately 21% oxygen. The reality is that our bodies need only a certain level of oxygen for optimum health and under normal circumstances, the amount in the air is ideal for our good health. Too little or too much oxygen can be equally harmful. Too little oxygen is technically called hypoxia. With too little oxygen our cells and tissues can literally starve and organs such as the brain become damaged. If the situation continues, organs can fail and we will eventually die.

Oxygen toxicity involves the other extreme of "dose," essentially too much oxygen. The two ways that oxygen toxicity can occur is by forcing it into our lungs at too high a pressure or forcing it into our lungs at too high a percentage over a long period of time. Oxygen toxicity affects the central nervous system (CNS), the lungs and the eyes. Which tissue is most likely to be affected depends upon whether the excess oxygen is at too high a pressure with a higher percentage than normal or whether it is at normal pressure but too high a percentage for a long period of time. It is possible to tolerate 100% oxygen for 24 to 48 hours at sea level. But problems can begin to arise after only a few hours, and the likelihood of severe tissue damage increases as time goes on.

Since the 19th century it has been known that breathing too high a concentration of oxygen for too long a period of time can produce toxicity. In reality, oxygen toxicity is more of a concern for premature newborns in neonatal care units, scuba divers and astronauts. How does this work?

Many premature babies have underdeveloped lungs. They lack lung proteins called surfactants that help to keep the lungs open so air can enter. Without assistance they would suffer from oxygen deficiency. They need oxygen delivered to the lungs and tissues at higher concentrations since their lungs are not mature enough to accomplish what is needed. This is usually performed in the hospital's Neonatal Intensive Care Unit (NICU). In these units, higher concentrations of oxygen can be delivered either via a hood (for babies who can breathe on their own) or though a mechanical ventilator, which helps to fill the collapsed lungs. The latter may also deliver oxygen under high pressure to help the babies breathe. But it is a fine art to provide just enough oxygen and not too much. Under these circumstances, oxygen toxicity can occur that alters lung development, immune system development and the vascular development of the eye. The latter scenario results in vision problems for the child.

Much of the damage caused by oxygen toxicity appears to come from the overproduction of oxygen free radicals and damage to the tissues. Breathing oxygen over 60% for too long can cause multiple problems. The eye is a vulnerable site because premature babies don't have complete blood system development to support the eye. Oxygen toxicity can interfere with and then alter the course of the needed vascular development.

In the case of scuba diving, oxygen is usually carried at either its normal concentration (21%) or at high concentrations for certain periods of time — called hyperbaric oxygen. However, as the diver moves to different depths, the external pressure increases. Diving too deep can cause the oxygen to be under too high a pressure, and toxic amounts can be delivered to the blood and tissues while breathing. The oxygen toxicity created can lead to seizures and brain damage.

For astronauts, breathing oxygen safely depends upon their situation. For example, they are able to safely breathe 100% oxygen for days in the orbiting capsule because the pressure in the capsule is only a fraction of what is found on earth. However, changes during space walks and re-entry mean that the pressure and the concentration of oxygen need to be adjusted to ensure the astronauts both avoid decompression and avoid a lack of oxygen or oxygen toxicity.

Of course, for most of our day-to-day encounters, the oxygen in the air is at a level that is safe, beneficial and required for life. This example with oxygen serves as a reminder that virtually any chemical or drug, even those required for life, can become toxic given a high enough concentration. For this reason, it is important for us to identify which concentrations of chemicals and drugs are safe for our children and which are potential problems for their health and well-being.

Selenium: Deficiency, Health (Immune Protection) and Toxicity

A good example of Paracelsus' idea can be found in our exposure to the mineral, selenium (designated as "Se" on the chemical periodic table). Selenium is an essential micronutrient that is involved with an enzyme (glutathione peroxidase) that is important in the detoxification processes to get rid of oxygen radicals. Glutathione peroxidases are a family of enzymes that, in effect, have antioxidant activity. They convert two dangerous chemicals to safer alternatives. These particular enzymes can take hydrogen peroxide and turn it into water, and they can take very dangerous lipid-radicals and make them into by-products that the body is able to handle. The trick is that the enzymes must have selenium in them to function. For this reason, one of the major roles of selenium is as an antioxidant. Selenium, through its role in glutathione peroxidase, helps to protect our tissues and organs from oxidative damage as our body fights infections and cancer.

Selenium is naturally found in many of the foodstuffs we eat such as cereals (e.g., oatmeal) and grains used to make bread. Selenium content in plants such as wheat is influenced by the soil content where the crop was grown, and this can vary widely. In fact even within the same country, soils in some areas can be deficient in selenium while soils in other regions may contain dangerously high levels of the mineral. At the extremes, this translates directly into the production of selenium-deficient wheat or selenium-toxic wheat depending upon the locale (an example of the latter is found in China). Many individuals also obtain selenium through the food chain (e.g., poultry and other meats) as well as via dietary supplements. This is important because selenium intake is needed for good health. Selenium has a unique antioxidant function that isn't covered by other antioxidants such as vitamin E and vitamin C. So if the level of selenium intake is too low, it results in disease.

Selenium deficiency can affect several different tissues and organs. It leads to diseases such as Keshan Disease, which is associated with an enlarged heart. The disease is given its name after Keshan province in China where the soil is deficient in selenium, and the crops grown locally do not provide sufficient amounts of selenium. Since its naming, the disease has been identified in other countries as well (e.g., New Zealand and Finland). Children and women are particularly susceptible to the disease. Once the heart muscle has been damaged from selenium deficiency, selenium supplementation does not reverse the damage.

In contrast, selenium toxicity, also called selenosis, produces symptoms such as gastrointestinal distress, hair loss, fatigue and neurological damage. Selenium toxicity has been found in certain areas of China where local corn grown in very high selenium soils was a major part of the diet.

As an anti-inflammatory agent, selenium may be important in combating inflammation-related conditions such as cardiovascular disease. Other investigators have reported that selenium levels may be important in certain autoimmune diseases such as autoimmune thyroiditis (Grave's disease and Hashimoto's disease).

Some Factors are Rarely Safe in Nature, Others are Rarely Dangerous

If the dose makes the poison, there are certainly chemicals and drugs that are dangerous at the concentration we usually encounter in nature. Table 1.1 shows a comparison of toxic doses for several chemicals and drugs.

The comparison of relative toxicity for sarin gas vs. vitamin A or for ricin toxin vs. diazepam is remarkable. It highlights the fact that some toxins are only theoretically safe and at the concentration we usually see in nature, they represent significant health hazards. One simply does not want to encounter the botulism toxin or ricin toxin outside of a medical clinic, since a little goes a long way in terms of potential harm to our health.

However, other chemicals and drugs are of little health concern at the levels we are likely to encounter in our daily lives. An example of the latter is amygdalin. This toxin is contained in apple seeds and in some fruit pits. When ingested and in the acid environment of the stomach, amygdalin is converted to cyanide. With enough cyanide, it can kill you. But you would have to eat several buckets full of apple seeds to ingest dangerous levels of amygdalin. So toxicity from amygdalin found in

Table 1.1. Sample adult toxicity of different chemicals (approximate single dose level of each chemical that is considered hazardous to a 170 lb adult).

Toxin	Dose	Toxin	Dose
Botulism toxin	0.4 micrograms	Cyanide	116 milligrams
Ricin	463 micrograms	Acetaminophen	12 grams
VX (nerve gas)	8 milligrams	Aspirin	23 grams
Sarin	15 milligrams	Vitamin A	>39 grams

Botulism toxin is more than 100 million times more toxic than Vitamin A for a single dose.

Note: This table is only provided to illustrate the magnitude of the differences for toxicity and should not be used as a personal safety guide.

apples is a theoretical possibility but not a practical danger. In contrast, many apricot pits contain enough amygdalin to be a practical problem. In the 1990s, some health food products that were imported into the United States were found to contain enough amygdalin-containing apricot pits in one bag to kill several people.

Children are Special in Toxicology

Our children have different safety concerns that must be distinguished from those of adults. They are not simply smaller versions of adults. The challenge for us as a society is that we have been far more successful at defining safe vs. harmful doses for adults than for the various developmental stages of a child's life. This needs to change.

Benefits and Risks of Aspirin: Children are Not Small Adults

Aspirin (or acetylsalicylic acid) would certainly qualify as one of the miracle drugs of the 20th century if not of human civilization. It has been mass-produced as a human therapeutic agent for over 100 years. Even before that, the bark of white willow trees (a source of a precursor to salicylic acid) was used by the ancient Greeks and Native Americans to treat pain. Yet, while it has tremendous potential benefits when used at moderate doses by most adults, safety for children is not simply a matter of lowering the adult dose of aspirin to fit a child's body weight. Instead, we now know that aspirin presents very specific age-related risks for children. Children are not simply smaller versions of adults.

Aspirin blocks the production of inflammatory metabolites called prostaglandins (produced by macrophages and other cells). These metabolites are involved in the chemical cascades that lead to pain and fever. By interfering with these cascades, aspirin is effective at reducing fever (antipyretic activity), alleviating pain (analgesic activity) and reducing the swelling (anti-inflammatory activity) associated with inflammatory reactions. A health risk to adults for consuming moderate doses of aspirin would be an allergic reaction to the drug. At higher levels, thinning of the stomach lining, ulcers, problems with blood clotting and kidney dysfunction are concerns. But the vast majority of adults benefit greatly from the moderate use of aspirin as demonstrated by decades of results.

Yet, this adult miracle drug has added health risks for some children. For children, aspirin presents the risk of Reye's syndrome particularly in children suffering from a fever. The condition connected to Reye's syndrome, as seen in aspirin-treated children from infants to teenagers, often looks similar to a viral illness such as meningitis including symptoms of vomiting, diarrhea and irritability. The actual mechanisms leading to Reye's syndrome are not well known, but mitochondrial toxicity may be involved. However, it is not known if it is a cause of organ damage or one of the effects.

Reye's syndrome is associated with liver degeneration and can lead to brain inflammation, damage and even death if left untreated. The liver problems appear to arise when enzyme activity changes and certain lipids get over-produced in the liver and flood the serum and other tissues. Excess glutamate appears to cause toxicity in the brain particularly to astrocytes (brain macrophages). While Reye's syndrome is relatively rare, it is an excellent example of the difference in health risks for adults as opposed to children. Because of the risk of Reye's syndrome, aspirin use is not recommended for individuals under 20 years of age.

Beyond the immediate uses of aspirin for treating headaches and fevers in adults, regular use of aspirin in adults can have multiple longer-term benefits. In fact, regular use of low dose aspirin is now recommended for middle-aged adults to reduce the risk of heart disease in men and stroke in women. This lesson of age-related risks for aspirin is one that we should apply to the entire spectrum of chemical and drug safety for children.

Understanding the dose and potential health risks can make the difference between a chemical, drug or dietary factor being safe and promoting good health or being toxic and damaging health. A significant amount of time and money has been invested in identifying the risk of environmental exposures relevant to adult populations. Ironically, despite the fact that our children represent our future, we know less about the safety of these factors for the developing immune and neurological systems of children than we do for ourselves.

Conclusions

The legacy of Paracelsus is that we appreciate the value of both natural and synthetic chemicals and drugs and the ways in which they may benefit health. But we also understand that even too much of an otherwise good thing can harm us. Knowing what is safe, what promotes our health and what impairs our health is the minimum of what toxicology can and should tell us. But toxicology has to be used to give us those answers. Safety testing when restricted to adults does little to help us protect our children. The lessons of children's special sensitivities, such as the recently discovered risk of Reye's syndrome, should guide us in the testing lab before medications are approved as safe for children. These lessons should not have to be learned in our homes.

Overview of Toxicology 101

- The motto of toxicology is: the dose makes the poison.
- Specific chemicals and drugs are not necessarily good or bad. But the doses of chemicals and drugs can be good or bad.
- Even too much of a good thing can be bad (e.g., oxygen at 100% can be toxic).
- Knowing what doses may harm children is our goal.
- Basic features of children (e.g., higher breathing rate) make them more sensitive to the environment
- An exposure that is safe for adults may not be safe for children.

Chapter 2 — What's the Risk?

Introduction

One of the reasons we wrote this book on strategies for reducing the risks for the child's immune system is because, at present in most countries, the risk of childhood immune dysfunction is significant, worrisome and, at least partly, unnecessary. So providing parents, families and physicians with information that could help them to better protect their child's immune system could help to reduce the incidence of illness and improve quality of life. But part of having this type of desired effect depends upon the actual risks involved in childhood immune dysfunction and how changes in day-to-day life and improved early-life safety testing of chemicals and drugs could help to reduce those risks.

Since reducing risk of immune dysfunction and related illness begins and ends with the idea of "risk," we need to take a moment to look more closely at that idea. This chapter will consider a series of five questions concerning risk. They are: What is risk? How does it relate to your child as an individual? How does risk involve the immune system and immune-related disease? What can we hope to gain by paying closer attention? What if we can't do it all?

What is Risk?

In this book, risk is the probability that your child will develop an environmentally-linked, immune-related disease or condition. The concern is specifically for your child. But the data used to determine the probability of risk for your child come from a wide variety of children who share similar genetic backgrounds and/or environmental experiences with your child. Therefore, it is only a probability and is likely to fall somewhere between the chance the sun will come up tomorrow (not 100% but close) and the chance that the authors of this book will win the next Powerball lottery (presently zero although it might be higher if we actually bought a ticket).

The first thing to realize is that health risk is virtually never zero and often it is not 100% either. It is somewhere in between 0 and 100. But that number matters and can dramatically affect our decisions. We accept some level of risk on a daily basis. But there is also risk we consciously refuse to accept. This past month an individual went over Niagara Falls with absolutely no protection. He survived. Were his chances of survival good based on the data? No. Would anyone recommend this as a nice vacation-spot activity? No. Most people die making the same attempt. In contrast, would people feel comfortable with a less rocky view of Niagara Falls, possibly by car to one of the parks that overlook the Falls? Yes. Hoards of people do and have survived to show their vacation pictures to family and friends — over and over again.

In a less dramatic way, we make health risk-based decisions virtually every day of our lives. When we go grocery shopping, the risk of buying tainted food on that day from that store that leads to hospitalization for salmonella poisoning is not zero. But it is small. In fact the number is so small in Western countries that it rarely stops us from shopping for food or eating. However, if we are on the way to the store and hear on the news that salmonella-contaminated spinach has led to multiple hospitalizations in the past 24 hours in our county, do we rush to the produce section of the store and decide to add a spinach salad to that evening's menu? Hopefully not. At a minimum, you probably want more information on the outbreak and would delay beginning that Popeye the Sailor diet for a few days. That original small "risk" number has now grown much larger. It has become a level of risk that you are probably unwilling to accept for either you or your family.

In this book, we attempt to give you the equivalent of that heads up to a salmonella outbreak. The factors we discuss are those that change the immune risk ball game for your child. That is why the more you know about the risks, the better chance you have of making informed decisions. Some factors are helpful and reduce risk such as the intake of moderate levels of antioxidants. Others are potentially harmful such as problematic exposures to lead or PCBs. Additionally, some things may be relatively easy to change (e.g., avoiding tobacco smoke). Others may be more difficult for some families (e.g., avoiding traffic pollution). But having the information available that allows you to identify the risk factors for your child is an important first step.

How Does Risk Apply to Your Child?

The more that is known about your child's environmental exposures and experiences (and genetic background), the more accurately one can predict the risk of immune dysfunction and immune-related disease. A lot is known. For example, if your child is raised in a household where both the mother and father smoke, the risk of your child developing asthma is increased by at least 30%. Does that mean that your child will develop asthma? No. Not every child will. But if your child is raised in a home with no tobacco smoke is the risk of asthma and airway disease significantly lower? Yes.

Another example of dealing with risk would be purchasing a car and trying to decide between two models as your options. For help with your decision, you are using the experiences and data collected from consumer groups on the performance and reliability of your two car model options in terms of how often those car models break down and need repairs. You might decide to go with the one consumers have reported as the more reliable option. If you purchase a top-rated car model that has outstanding consumer feedback as to reliability, does that mean your new car is guaranteed not to break down or be a lemon? No. If you are very unlucky, you might get the one in a million car of that model in that year that missed a critical assembly line part and has chronic repair problems. In contrast, if you buy a car that ranks among the poorest for reliability based on consumer experience, is it certain you will be spending more time in the repair shop than on the road? Not necessarily. You could be exceptionally lucky. But most customers who bought that car model were not. So you might want to have your credit card ready and the repair shop on speed dial once you leave the dealer's lot.

In this day and time, most people would not think of buying a car without knowing something about the benefits (e.g., I can afford it now and it seats everyone in the family) and risks (e.g., Will it still be running in three years and can I afford to fuel it then?) of that purchase.

How Does Risk Relate to the Developing Immune System and Immune-Related Disease?

Our children have a certain risk of developing immune problems and immune-related disease over their lifetime, and one we will argue is unnecessarily high. Table 2.1 shows the recent prevalence of immune-related diseases based on data collected from developed countries (primarily U.S., U.K., Continental Europe).

Table 2.1. Prevalence of immune-based diseases.

Immune/Inflammatory-Based Disease or Condition	Approximate Range of Prevalence % (US/UK/Continental Europe)
Recurrent Otitis Media	18–26
Childhood Asthma	15–25
Atopic Dermatitis	15
Pediatric Allergic Rhinitis	8–12
Pediatric Food Allergy	5–7
Childhood Type 1 Diabetes	0.2
Childhood Leukemia	0.1
Autoimmune Thyroid Diseases (all ages)	2–7
Atherosclerosis (all ages)	1.7
Rheumatoid Arthritis (all ages)	1.0
Celiac Disease (all ages)	0.8
Lupus (all ages)	0.2
Inflammatory Bowel Disease (all ages)	0.2
Chronic Fatigue Syndrome (all ages)	0.2
Multiple Sclerosis (all ages)	0.1
Metabolic Syndromes/Disorders	**

Adapted from Dietert RR, Zelikoff JT. Pediatric immune dysfunction and health risks following early-life immune insult. *Curr Pediatr Rev* 5(1): 36–51, 2009.

**Note that certain metabolic disorders are thought to have misregulated inflammation as an underlying basis of the condition.

If one examines the totals, even considering that some individuals will develop more than one of these diseases, it is clear that approximately 25%–50% of children are likely to face at least one immune-related disease during their lifetime. Many of these diseases (e.g., childhood asthma, type 1 diabetes) have increased in prevalence since the 1960s. Our known environmental factors account for only a portion of this increase. This suggests we are not identifying all the risk factors causing immune dysfunction with our current testing requirements, and that an excellent opportunity exists to reduce the risk for our children.

Where risk factors have been identified (e.g., tobacco smoke, alcohol, dioxin, antibiotics), each one has the potential to cause childhood immune dysfunction. In some cases, exposure to these toxins increases sensitivity to other toxins. This has been reported for exposure to the metals, arsenic and lead. For this reason, avoiding exposure to known toxins and conditions that are likely to damage the developing immune system can go a long way toward reducing the risk for later-life immune dysfunction and the associated diseases. For a particular child, no single preventative action of avoiding a toxin or taking an antioxidant supplement can absolutely guarantee that his or her immune system never has a problem. But it can minimize the risk for immune problems and help your family stay out of that tainted spinach aisle.

What Can We Hope to Gain Through Reduced Risk?

The information that is provided in later chapters is prioritized based on the likelihood your child might be exposed to an environmental factor or condition and the magnitude of the effect that factor produces (positive or negative effect on the developing immune system). We have avoided trying to provide actual risk numbers for each environmental factor such as "exposure to tobacco smoke increases the risk of childhood asthma by _X_%." The reason for this is because different studies have reported different numbers even if they all agree on the nature, direction and significance of the toxin-induced change. Our goal is to make the information as useful and accessible as possible. Long lists of numbers may not help to achieve this. Instead, we have tried to reflect the magnitude of immune health concern for each factor in our prioritization guide (e.g., the Top 25 List).

There is one basic reason why reduction of risk for immune dysfunction should be an important priority for parents. Most of the diseases linked with Developmental Immunotoxicity (DIT) and immune dysfunction are chronic diseases that require a lifetime of medical treatment and prescription drugs. They impact quality of life for the child's entire life, as well as place a financial burden on the family. The benefits of disease prevention and avoidance for your child greatly outweigh the costs of life-long medical treatment for chronic disease. For example, just think about the need for medical treatment, impact on daily life and additional later life disease risks that are associated with immune-related diseases such as type 1 diabetes, celiac disease, atherosclerosis, arthritis, multiple sclerosis and asthma.

What If We Can't Do It All?

Subsequent chapters in this book include a significant list of "do's" and "don'ts" to guide parents in decisions and steps for supporting the development of their child's immune system. As previously mentioned, some of these steps are likely to be relatively easy and should require little if any change in daily routine. Other changes might require a bit more forethought but are still very achievable goals. However, most parents are likely to find at least some items on the lists that are frustrating at best and would be heroic accomplishments at a minimum. Not everyone need be elected mayor or president to institute all the changes before starting with the easy ones. Each problematic toxin avoided and positive dietary factor added to the menu is a step in right direction. Each one tilts the odds more in favor of your child's immune system developing correctly. The most important consideration is to use those prenatal and postnatal windows of immune vulnerability to a health advantage rather than ignoring them and risking later-life regrets. Doing it all is not needed. Doing something is likely to be a gift that will grow in appreciation for years to come.

Overview of What's the Risk?

- Zero risk rarely, if ever, exists when it comes to health decisions.
- We already make decisions every day involving health risk (e.g., of injury when we step of our bed). So this is nothing new.
- Informed decisions involving health risks are likely to be more helpful for our children.
- Sorting out the no-brainer decisions from the closer calls for your child's immune system is what this book is about.

Chapter 3 — The Risk Exercises

Introduction

In Chapter 1, we talked about toxicology and the importance of dose in determining if an exposure to a chemical or drug presents a danger for our children. We then talked about risk and how it can influence our daily decisions. This mini-chapter builds upon the toxicology and risk concepts by providing two exercises that demonstrate how our personal ideas about potential health risk can affect our decisions. We hope you find them to be instructive and possibly a little entertaining.

Identifying Your Comfort Zone for Risks

Some exposures, like strolling through a burning building, are truly dangerous, and no one has to tell us they are dangerous. Some are helpful and may be obvious as well, such as making sure to eat a nutritious breakfast everyday. Some exposures are dangerous but the danger is not yet known, like wading into a river without knowing where the drop-offs are. In that event, we are unlikely to do anything since we are unaware of the danger. We lack the needed information.

Each of these decisions is comparatively easy.

Where it gets interesting and challenging is when there is a gray area. Associated with a particular exposure or activity there may be both some level of risk but perhaps also some benefit or convenience. Some exposures may have a degree of uncertainty as far as toxic danger goes, but they aren't worth the risk because the potential for serious danger is too great (e.g., preparing your first dinner of poisonous blowfish with no prior instruction). A majority of environmental exposures are relatively safe as long as the exposure is in moderation (e.g., recommended dose of Tylenol for adults). But then there is the new drug that may help with a condition, but has a list of side effects as long as your arm (just listen to some drug ads on TV). Will the drug help? Are you among those who will have serious side effects? When are you comfortable with the benefit vs. the risk? When are you not?

This book will spend comparatively less time on the toughest gray areas than on the clearer options. It will focus on the known and suspected toxins for the immune system and on those gray areas where the potential for danger appears to be significantly increased over the benefits of ignoring the potential risks. But in the end, many of the decisions that parents will make after consulting their physicians will involve their own comfort zone for risk and in this case, risk for toxicity to the developing immune system. The more age-relevant toxicology information that is available to parents and physicians, the clearer those decisions are likely to be. That information may help to reduce the number of gray areas that parents encounter for their child's immune system.

Exercise 1. The Snake in the Grass Exercise

If you want to begin to examine the area of toxicology, risk and comfort zones, here is a thought exercise. Its purpose is to remind you of the types of decisions concerning risks you already make.

It is a lovely spring day and you are out preparing your garden beds for those young plants and seeds. Your child runs up to report he/she has seen a snake around the backyard compost pile. Certainly, it is something that warrants your attention as a parent from the standpoint of safety. We know that some snakes are poisonous and through their bite they can inject toxins into our bodies. Others are not poisonous and are unlikely to bite under most circumstances. However, some parents may not want their child anywhere near any snakes that are on the loose regardless of the type of snake. That's an individual choice. But the more information available, the easier the decision is likely to be.

So in this exercise, you as the parent go check out the snake.

Option A — The "snake" is not a snake but rather a large earthworm. The earthworm is happy in the compost pile and is helping to break down the materials. There is benefit in the earthworm's presence and little downside. You take the opportunity to broaden you child's knowledge of animal diversity (earthworms vs. snakes) and go back to your gardening knowing your child is safe, and you are likely to have some decent natural fertilizer later in the summer.

Option B — There is a snake but it is relatively small and a species that is both non-aggressive and non-poisonous (e.g., garter snakes). You remembered seeing mice around your compost pile the prior weekend. The snake is there for the buffet. This is closer to a gray area and tests your evaluation of potential risks to your family (from a bite) vs. the benefits of having the snake reduce the backyard rodent population. The scale may tip depending upon your evaluations of the snake's size and nature and the age of your child. Alternatively, you may not like the idea of snakes of any kind in your backyard, period, and will deal with the rodents in another way. This decision may go either way and is likely to depend upon information as well as your comfort zone.

Option C — Your child is correct. There is a snake and it is a poisonous pit viper with a nasty disposition. This is a rather clear danger to any and all. Benefits aren't likely to be in your thoughts at this time. You and your child go into the house, and you call animal control with the appropriate information.

Just as Option A is an easy decision. Option C is as well. But it is made easy by the knowledge that there's a good chance either you or your child could get bitten and poisoned. Information in this book will inform parents of those well-established toxins for the developing immune system.

To make this an actual exercise, specify the type and size of different non-poisonous snakes for Option B and decide your course of action for each case. For example, the snake could be a:

1) 8″ long garter snake,
2) 12″ long rat snake,

3) 20″ long Western Hognose snake (known for repeated biting defenses),
4) 36″ long boa snake.

There is no right and no wrong answer. It is a matter of personal choice.

Exercise 2. Metallica-Unplugged

You are a pregnant woman and have just learned you are heading to dinner with a group from work to host business visitors from out of town. The restaurant is a local sushi bar. Normally you like sushi. But you remember from this book and other sources that both mercury and PCB contamination of larger fish species such as tuna are major immune and neurological health concerns particularly for the developing baby. You also know that omega-3 fatty acids from fish can be helpful for developing babies.

Once at the restaurant you:

Option A — Load your plate with the full array of tuna items you used to enjoy reminding yourself of the benefits of omega-3 fatty acids.

Option B — Take half the amount of the tuna offerings you would normally enjoy and sample more of the vegetable-based items for the other half of your dinner.

Option C — Shun all items made with larger species of fish and eat other menu choices.

Again, there is no inherently right or wrong answer. You are weighing lots of information. How much mercury exposure for the baby is too much? Does eating omega-3 fatty acids tonight outweigh the risk of mercury and PCBs? Can you find menu alternatives you can eat beyond the tuna?

These are real life decisions and there will be many more for parents to make. The information in this book and other resources should assist parents as they weigh these types of decisions. Similar risk-based health decisions will pertain to virtually every stage of a child's life.

Overview of the Risk Exercises

- Risk exercises may help your awareness of the safety-related decisions you are already making.
- Many of the suggested strategies presented later in this book are not difficult or challenging. Do the easy ones first before tackling the harder ones.
- Some immune-related decisions may be 50:50 options. In those cases, your gut instinct may lead you to the better option.

Chapter 4 — Introduction to the Immune System

Your child's immune system has two primary functions: (1) to protect against foreign invaders (e.g., viruses and bacteria) and cancer cells and (2) to maintain the balanced function (called homeostasis) of your tissues and organs. To carry out these functions it is necessary for the immune system to station cells in virtually every part of your child's body. They are constantly surveying the body for potential problems. Here, the immune cells act like a personal army, searching out foreign invaders and tumor cells in order to destroy them. They also remove dead body cells without causing damage to healthy cells (i.e., no inflammation should occur). Immune cells are the police force of every tissue and organ. When they function properly, your child's tissues are more likely to function properly as well.

In carrying out these functions, the immune system has the capacity to: (1) learn, (2) remember and (3) mobilize cells that seek and destroy specific invaders. The immune system is complex as it is composed of many different types of cells (generally known as white blood cells or leukocytes) that work together to protect your child. Each cell type has different tasks, and they coordinate with each other to better protect your child.

To properly introduce you to your child's immune system, we will look at how the immune system responds in the case of six different children. Through these children's cases, you will learn the names of the cells and the chemicals they secrete that provide your child with important immune protection from disease.

Case #1. Tyrone's Tiff Against Tetanus —

Topics — Acquired Immunity, Humoral Immunity, Antibody (Immunoglobulin) Production, Booster Vaccinations

Tetanus is a life-threatening disease. It affects nerves, essentially paralyzes muscles and is produced by the *Clostridium* bacteria. When present in the environment, this toxin-containing bacteria can invade open wounds and within a few days the toxin can reach dangerous levels. Vaccinations beginning in childhood and continuing into adulthood provide effective protection against the disease. Tyrone is a five-year-old who loves to climb and explore, but he invariably collects scrapes and scratches and today is one of those days. Tyrone stepped on a rusty nail and has a puncture wound. Fortunately, he received one of his series of childhood vaccinations (tetanus) only last month. The injection (often a mixture of tetanus toxoid and other vaccines as well), contains a safe (inactivated) form of the *Clostridium* toxin whose active form causes the disease (also called "lockjaw"). Tyrone's **dendritic cells** and **macrophages** took up the toxin and displayed it (presented it) to B and **T lymphocytes**. Those able to respond started an **acquired immune response**. The **B lymphocytes** had developed in the bone marrow while most T lymphocytes developed in the thymus. The latter come in several forms: (1) those that help immune responses **T helper cells (Ths)**, those that regulate what responses are permitted **T regulatory cells (Tregs)**, and those that carry out responses **cytotoxic T lymphocytes (CTLs)**.

The acquired immune response that now protects Tyrone from the toxin is the production of circulating **antibodies (also called immunoglobulins)** by B lymphocytes. It developed as a result of the series of vaccinations he received and will continue to protect Tyrone for several more years. Because the needed B lymphocytes cloned themselves many times over after Tyrone's vaccination, they were able to make lots of immunoglobulin(Ig) against the tetanus toxin. That cloning process by B and T lymphocytes is a hallmark of the acquired (also called adaptive) immune response.

Most of the antibodies that are produced are a type of **immunoglobulin** called **G (IgG)**, which is the predominant antibody found in blood. IgG comes in several forms that are adapted to our needs. Some forms cross the placenta to help the fetus. Other forms of IgG interact with macrophages and immune cells to recruit them in our defense. Other types of immunoglobulins are also made by B lymphocytes **(IgM, IgD, IgA, IgE)**. These are well suited for other needs. Antibody molecules can work directly against viruses, bacteria and toxins. But they also can work with various leukocytes (macrophages, **natural killer (NK) cells**, **basophils**, **eosinophils** and **mast cells**) to attack pathogens. Periodic booster vaccinations against the tetanus toxoid (about every ten years) will continue to protect Tyrone throughout his life.

Case #2. Frank Fights the Flu —

Topics — Acquired Immunity, Cell-Mediated Immunity, T Helper 1 Immune Responses, Cytotoxic T Lymphocytes, Cytokines, Interleukins, Free Radicals

Six-year-old Frank missed getting a flu vaccination this year, and he has just been exposed to the influenza virus while at the local shopping mall with his mother. The virus targets the epithelial cells lining the airways. If the virus gets by protective barriers such as the nasal hairs, it can set up home in the epithelial cells. Frank's immune system will mount an **acquired immune response** involving both B and T lymphocytes. If Frank's immune system has not seen this particular virus before, it will take several days for the flu-specific lymphocytes to appear.

Immune cells called **dendritic cells** get the immune response party started by displaying (called presenting) parts of the flu virus to the B and T lymphocytes. They also secrete immune system hormones. These are generally called **cytokines** or sometimes **interleukins (meaning between leukocytes). Interleukins are designated by IL-followed by a number designation (e.g., IL-1, IL-2,...)**. These immune hormones ramp up specific types of immune responses and also help to promote or dampen-down inflammation. When the dendritic cells present part of the flu virus and also secrete cytokines, the **B lymphocytes (also called B cells)** that develop will contribute to **humoral immunity (meaning involving soluble proteins like antibodies)**. B cells will produce antibodies (also called immunoglobulins) found in fluids (in this case in the airways). The antibodies will try to clear the virus. But in this case they are usually not effective since the virus hides out inside cells.

Instead, it is the other arm of **acquired immunity**, called **cell-mediated immunity (meaning that immune cells directly attack and kill the virus-infected cells)**, that will give Frank protection from the virus. T lymphocytes are produced specific for the flu virus. These are called cytotoxic T lymphocytes, and they can directly attack virus-infected cells killing them before the virus can spread further. These T cells get made when a **T helper 1 (Th1)** type of acquire immune response is produced. Other immune cells called **macrophages** and **neutrophils (usually more important in bacterial infections)** try to help by producing **oxygen radicals** (a type of **free radical**) as well as **nitric oxide** to kill the virus. They may also make **prostaglandins** using the fatty acids on their cell surfaces. But these products can also cause tissue damage in the process. In fact, one of the risks from flu for children and the elderly is if the airway tissue damage is too great and cannot be fully repaired. Too much inflammation is not helpful.

The cell-mediated response is effective and after a period of illness including fever caused by certain macrophage-produced **cytokines**, Frank recovers. Of course by next year the flu strain is likely to have changed so Frank's very specific, long-term acquired immunity may or may not protect him again. That is why more frequent vaccination is recommended for flu.

Case #3. Susie's Sniffles and Sneezes —

Topics — Acquired Immunity, Humoral Immunity, T Helper 2 Immune Responses, Immunoglobulin E (IgE), Eosinophils, Basophils

Twelve-year-old Susie is getting ready for a big soccer match when she awakens on a sunny May morning to a sneezing fit and nasal congestion. She also notices that her itchy eyes look bloodshot. It could be a cold, but unlike her usual colds, there is no fever nor even a sore throat. In fact, it is her first experience with allergic rhinitis (also commonly known as hayfever).

The burst of flowering trees in the area has provided lots of pollen, and Susie's immune system thinks (inappropriately) that is something harmful. It saw oak pollen the prior spring when the **dendritic cells** presented it to B and T cells. The B cells made a special type of antibody called **immunoglobulin E (IgE)**. Ironically, this antibody is really good at fighting against parasitic worms. The problem is that the oak pollen is not a dangerous parasite.

As with other antibodies, IgE gets produced by B lymphocytes. In this **acquired immune response**, **T helper 2 (Th2) cells** direct the B lymphocytes to make IgE instead of a different antibody that would not cause allergic symptoms. The sneezing begins when other immune cells (called **mast cells**) located around the blood vessels in Susie's nose have IgE coating their surfaces. When the oak pollen lands on these cells, they release **histamine** and the sneezing begins. Other immune cells, **eosinophils** and **basophils (called granulocytes because they contain grainy-looking sacs of enzymes inside)**, can also get into the action by releasing inflammation-producing chemicals and increasing the nasal and eye swelling and irritation. An additional concern is that hayfever can sometimes progress to later-life asthma or other allergic conditions. A misdirected Th2-driven acquired immune response is the part of the immune system involved in this condition.

Case #4. Carlos Cancels Cancer —

Topics — Innate Immunity, Natural Killer (NK) Cells, Protection Against Cancer

Carlos is an active seven-year-old who, along with his parents, never knew his immune system successfully fought cancer cells today. A small number of cancerous cells developed in his liver. But immune cells responsible for constantly surveying the body for cancer (and virus-infected cells) detected them and killed them today. These lymphocytes are called **Natural Killer (NK) cells**, and they are part of the early response system called **innate immunity**.

Innate immunity can respond in minutes to hours while acquired immunity takes days to weeks for a response. Innate immunity does not require B lymphocytes with their antibodies or cytotoxic T lymphocytes (featured in acquired immune responses). Instead, as part of innate immunity, **NK cells** act directly by detecting subtle changes on the cancer cell surfaces that send up an immediate red flag. **NK cells are programmed to kill anything with abnormal cell surfaces** and let the rest of the immune system ask questions later. NK cells protect us from a small number of cancer cells on a regular basis. It is only if and when the small number of cancerous cells slips through the NK defense and multiplies further that acquired immunity gets involved.

Case #5. Sara's Splinter —

Topics — Innate Immune Responses, Macrophages, Neutrophils

Sara is an 11-year-old softball player on the neighborhood travel team. She just returned from a game having played in the outfield and scored a run. While on the bench, she picked up a wood splinter in one of her fingers. Splinters are common foreign objects for children and adults alike. Like all foreign objects (e.g., viruses, bacteria, diesel exhaust particles), once they have significant contact with our tissues, the immune system gets interested.

Neutrophils and **macrophages (cells that like to ingest or eat small invaders, a process called phagocytosis)** are often the first cells to arrive on the scene when tissue injury is involved (even if minor). If the injury involves bacteria, neutrophils are very important in killing and/or removing the bacteria. If the main threat is not from bacteria, macrophages are likely to be more important at the scene.

In this case, the splinter is much larger than a single virus or bacterium. Macrophages will surround the splinter and **wall it off**. This is why **callous areas** can develop if splinters remain in a finger for a very long time. Ironically, the same type of macrophage response can occur when lung macrophages encounter the bacteria that cause tuberculosis. But in that case, walling off large sections of the lungs creates a problem. It reduces the effectiveness of lung function.

In the case of Sara's finger with the splinter, the macrophages will help to wall off the splinter and will gradually pressure the splinter toward the surface. Hopefully, Sara's mother or father will give the macrophages a little extra help in removing the splinter.

Case #6. Tina Tackles a Tummy Ache —

Topics — Mucosal Immunity, Immunoglobulin A (IgA), Intraepithelial Lymphocytes (IELs), Gut-Associated Lymphoid Tissue (GALT)

Six-year-old Tina just enjoyed her favorite lunch, chicken salad. She also just avoided a tummy ache and potentially more serious G.I. distress. What Tina and her parents never knew is that a few pathogenic bacteria that love the G.I. tract were hiding among some of the lettuce leaves and were fully prepared to cause Tina health problems. But Tina had several lines of immune defense that form what is known as **mucosal immunity** (the immunity of tissues where mucus is produced).

Because Tina's immune system had seen this bacterium before, she already had antibodies to attack it that were perfectly designed for various secretions (saliva, tears, airway and G.I. tract fluids). These antibodies are called **Immunoglobulin A (IgA)**, and they are present in Tina's saliva. The IgA in Tina's saliva can keep many bacteria from ever reaching the stomach. If any bacteria make it past her stomach acids, her natural gut flora could help block their attachment to the gut lining.

Flow of mucus could help cleanse the gut of the invading bacteria. Also, specialized G.I. tract immune cells called **intraepithelial lymphocytes (IELs)** help to identify friendly bacteria from foes. The combined defense of the G.I. tract is often called **gut-associated lymphoid tissue or GALT**. In another mucosal immune tissue, the lung, there is also a respiratory counterpart to the GALT. In this case it is called **bronchus-associated lymphoid tissue or BALT**.

The prior six cases involve all the major cell types of the immune system. We will be mentioning these cells, their cytokines and their by-products (metabolites) repeatedly throughout this book. The following chart shows the immune cells organized into the most commonly used categories.

Major Cells of the Immune System

Leukocytes

- Lymphoid Cells
  - o B Lymphocytes
  - o T Lymphocytes
    - — T Helper Cells
    - — TRegs
    - — Cytoxic T Cells
  - o Natural Killer Cells
- Myeloid Cells
  - o Monocytes (a form of macrophage found only in the blood)
    - — Macrophages (former monocytes that have entered the tissues)
    - — Dendritic Cells
  - o Neutrophils
  - o Basophils
  - o Eosinophils
  - o Mast Cells

How Innate and Acquired Immunity Work Together

Innate and acquired immunity provide your child with an effective one-two punch against possible infections. Innate immunity is fast, but in general it is not very specific in terms of the invading virus or bacterium. In contrast, acquired (or adaptive) immunity is much slower than the innate response, but it is very specific to the virus or bacterium that infects your child. Additionally, acquired immunity has many different ways to attack the microbe (e.g., several different types of immunglobulins can be produced as well as cytotoxic T lymphocytes). Even when innate immunity does not completely clear an infection, it often gives your child much-needed time to make antibodies and T lymphocytes tailored for successfully attacking the microbe.

Innate vs. Acquired Immunity

- Innate immunity —
  - — rapid fire, front line of defense against infections and cancer
  - — mobilized by macrophages, neutrophils and natural killer cells
  - — no cell division needed to start an innate immune response
  - — more general than acquired immunity
  - — may produce more collateral damage of tissues
  - — lacks immunological memory

- Acquired/Adaptive immunity —
  - — involves B and/or T lymphocytes which must be cloned to fight the disease challenge
  - — specific for the pathogen or tumor cell antigen
  - — takes longer to develop
  - — is more intense the second time the same response is triggered (has immunological memory)

In the upcoming chapters, we will discuss how the immune system develops, what happens to it during pregnancy, and how a well functioning immune system can protect your child. We will also describe what happens when the developing immune system is damaged and becomes dysfunctional in the child. Because the immune system is so pivotal to good health and well-being, its care is an integral part of the overall care of your child.

Summary

- The immune system is one of the most important systems for long term health and well-being.
- Many different types of cells make up the immune system. Some are mobile and can move about your body. Immune cells are found in virtually every tissue and organ of the body.

- The immune system has both a front line defense strategy (innate immunity) and longer term very specific defense option (acquired immunity).
- Immune responses differ depending upon the type of disease challenge (e.g., virus vs. bacteria vs. parasite).
- The immune system can remember if it saw a particular pathogen before.
- A well-functioning immune system promotes good health. A dysfunctional immune system can, by itself, cause disease.

Chapter 5 — How the Immune System Develops

The immune system very well may be the second most complex system in the body (just behind the neurological system). Because it does as much to keep the body operating smoothly as it does to attack and destroy invading pathogens, it has a huge task that requires constant vigilance. Given this, it comes as no surprise that the immune system takes time to develop and fully mature. In general, it is not until the last stages of adolescence that all aspects of a child's immune system reach their full adult capacity. This means that childhood and adolescence are immunologically formative years.

However, the most important developmental events occur during pregnancy and the baby's first few years, a topic we'll also discuss in chapters 6 to 8. Most, if not all, of the developmental stages that occur during pregnancy are critical to ensuring that the immune system, and in fact the entire body, develops normally and is capable of protecting and maintaining good health for the next near century. Almost all of these stages never occur again at any other time in an individual's life. These are one-time events and as such are very critical and sensitive.

The following table shows how the immune system develops in parallel with the baby's body. It outlines what happens inside the womb from conception through birth. Week-by-week through each trimester, the table follows the course of your developing child's immune system and shows how important each step is to your child's lifelong health.

Gestational Development

Weeks/ General	General	Weeks/ Immune	Immune
1–2	— Conception and creation of the zygote — Journey through the fallopian tube to uterus — Cell division to form the blastocyst — Blastocyst embeds in the uterine wall (day 6–12) — Beginning of the embryonic stage	1–2	— Stem cells for the immune system including those that will produce macrophages and dendritic cells form in the yolk sac and one other area of the embryo
3	— Development of the brain, spinal cord, heart and GI tract		
4–5	— Arm and leg buds are visible — Heart is beating in a steady rhythm — Placenta beginning to form and is producing hormones. Rudimentary blood moves through the main blood vessels — Early structures form for the eyes and ears — Brain develops into five areas — Embryo = ¼ inch long	4–7	— Macrophage-like cells and dendritic cells emerge from the yolk sac — They begin to move to and take up residence in all the tissues and organs of the embryo's body. This process is called SEEDING. For example, some macrophages appear in the brain beginning at this time — Macrophages and dendritic cells are also found in the embryo's connective tissues
		5.5–7	— The liver becomes the center of blood/ immune cell creation

(*Continued*)

(*Continued*)

Weeks/ General	General	Weeks/ Immune	Immune
6	— Formation of lungs, jaw, nose and palate — Hand and feet buds have webbing that will become fingers and toes — Audible heartbeat heard on vaginal ultrasound — Embryo = ½ inch long	6	— Dendritic cells present in the rudimentary thymus, intestines and epidermis — Thymic stroma (structural thymus matrix) forms
		6.5	— Langerhans cells (a type of dendritic cell) are detected in the skin
7	— Every essential organ has begun to form — Embryo weighs less than an aspirin — Hair and nipple follicles are forming — Eyelids and tongue have begun to form — Elbows and toes are more visible — Trunk begins to straighten out	7	— Macrophages with molecules to display antigens to T cells appear in the liver
8	— Ears continue forming both inside and outside — Everything present in an adult is now present in the embryo — Bones are beginning to form — Muscles contract — Facial features are maturing — Eyelids are more developed	8	— Cells that will become T cells leave the liver and seed the thymus — Cells that will become B cells appear in the liver and part of the abdomen

(*Continued*)

(Continued)

Weeks/ General	General	Weeks/ Immune	Immune
	— **This ends the embryonic period** — Fetal period begins — Fetus = 1 inch long; size of a bean		
		8	— Gut associated lymphoid tissue (GALT) is first identified
		8–12	— Lymph nodes appear
9–13	— Genetalia are clearly male or female — The eyelids close — Fetus is able to make a fist — Buds for baby teeth appear — The head = ½ the size of the entire fetus — Fetus = 3 inches long; weighs 1 oz	9–12	— Thymocytes populate the thymus
		10	— Spleen appears — IgG and IgM antibodies are made in the spleen
		10–11	— Tonsils appear
		10–12	— The spleen starts participating in immune cell production — Surface IgM apparent on liver B cells
		10–16	— Immune stem cells migrate to the bone marrow

(Continued)

(*Continued*)

Weeks/ General	General	Weeks/ Immune	Immune
		11	— Cells in the thymus undergo gene rearrangements needed to produce T lymphocytes — IgE antibodies are created in the lungs and liver
		11–12	— Immune cell production shifts permanently to the bone marrow
		11–13	— Macrophages with molecules for displaying antigens appear in the lymph nodes
		11–15	— Peyer's patches develop in the gut (another site of B cell development) — The appendix, which creates and houses good gut bacteria, develops
		11–16	— The first time fetal lymphocytes are able to recognize and respond to cells from other individuals — If fetal organs were used in transplants, they would now be rejected by mature immune systems

(*Continued*)

(*Continued*)

Weeks/ General	General	Weeks/ Immune	Immune
		12	— Thymus begins to divide into two parts, the cortex and the medulla — Thymus lymphocytes undergo cell division when exposed to certain stimuli (a process called proliferation) — B cells detected in peripheral blood
		13	— Surface IgD antibody is first detected on liver B cells
		13–14	— Thymus lymphocytes become able to receive external signals from other cells that stimulate them to proliferate
		13–23	— B cells are now found in the spleen
14–16	— Fetal skin is transparent — Fine hair (lanugo) forms on the head — Fetus begins sucking and swallows bits of amniotic fluid — Fingerprints now developed on the tiny fingers — Meconium is now made in the GI tract — Mother may now feel flutters in abdomen from fetal movement — Sweat glands have developed — Liver and pancreas produce fluid secretions — Fetus = 6 inches long; weighs 4 oz	14	— Thymic medulla (the inner portion of the thymus) now has more macrophages and dendritic cells and fewer lymphocytes than does the cortex. Thymocytes move from the outer cortex into the inner cortex and then into the medulla as they mature

(*Continued*)

(*Continued*)

Weeks/ General	General	Weeks/ Immune	Immune
		14–16	— Major increase in the number of T cells
		14–1 yr	— Intraepithelial lymphocytes (IELs) emerge and enter the mucosal linings of the GI and reproductive tracts where they're housed (IELs that protect the gut)
		16–17	— Macrophages with molecules for displaying antigens appear in the thymic medulla
		16–19	— Spleen lymphocytes respond to antigens
		16–20	— B cells become abundant in the bone marrow
		16–38	— Macrophages are altered by the surfactants (proteins) made in the lungs
		16–2 yrs	— Astrocytes (a type of brain macrophage) first appear and then expand in the brain
17–20	— Mother feels movements more easily — Eyebrows, eyelashes, fingernails and toenails grow — Fetal skin produces vernix to cover and protect it from amniotic fluid — Fetal heartbeat heard through a stethoscope — Fetus = 8 inches long; weighs 12oz	17	— Thymic medulla fully formed — Primary lymph nodes develop — Kupffer cells (specialized macrophages) appear in the liver
		17–18	— IgG and IgM reach maximum amounts

(*Continued*)

(*Continued*)

Weeks/ General	General	Weeks/ Immune	Immune
		18	— Blood lymphocytes respond to antigens
		20	— Immune cell production permanently shifts from the liver to the bone marrow
21–23	— Lanugo covers the entire fetus — Fetus beginning to look like a newborn — Skin less transparent — Fat develops — Eyes are completely developed — Liver and pancreas are completing their development — Lower airways in the fetus' lungs develop — Fetus = 10–11 inches; weighs 1–1 ¼ pounds		
24–26	— Fetus now has sleep/wake cycles that mother is aware of — Startle reflexes begin — Lung air sacs begin forming — Brain begins a rapid development phase — Nervous system is sufficiently developed to control some functions — Fetus = 14 inches long; weighs 2 ¼ pounds		
25–28	— Brain develops rapidly — Respiratory system is sufficiently developed for some gas exchange — Nervous system controls some bodily functions		

(*Continued*)

(*Continued*)

Weeks/ General	General	Weeks/ Immune	Immune
27–32	— Fetus fills out and stores fat on its body — Some rhythmic breathing movement detected — Bones fully develop though they're still soft — Fetus stores its own calcium, iron and phosphorus — Eyelids open for the first time since the first trimester — Fetus = 15–17 inches long; weighs 4–4 ½ pounds	28	— Natural killer cells capable of functioning develop in the thymus
33–36	— Fetus moves into a head-down position getting ready for birth — Begins rapid weight gain — Lanugo disappears from the skin — Fetus becomes less red and wrinkly — Fetus = 16-19 inches long; weighs 5 ¾–6 ¾ pounds	36–1 yr	— The immune system's overall ability to respond to specific antigens (immunocompetence) **begins** to mature
		36–2 yrs	— Dendritic cells mature to promote a Th1 response as well as the fetal-established Th2 response. Both are needed

(*Continued*)

(Continued)

Weeks/ General	General	Weeks/ Immune	Immune
37–40	— 38 weeks is considered full term — Ready to make its appearance at any time — Fetal movement is reduced because it takes up most of the uterus with no space left over — Fingernails have grown long enough that they'll need to be cut shortly after birth — Breast buds visible on both sexes — Mother is supplying the fetus with antibodies — All organs are developed — Lungs will continue to develop until delivery — Hair on the head is now coarse and thick — Baby = 19–21 inches long; weighs 6 ¾–10 pounds		
	Postnatal	1–18 yrs	— Immune system memory for infectious agents such as bacteria and viruses becomes established and grows

Summary

The table comparing the timeline of immune development and general development of the baby illustrates an important point: there is no window of time during a pregnancy when a baby can afford to have its developing immune system disrupted. Different weeks of development involve different immune events in the maturation of the immune system. By scanning the table you can see that a toxic exposure at different times of the pregnancy would be likely to have different effects on the baby's immune system. Different events are happening almost every week. Because novel changes are happening to the immune system throughout pregnancy, no part of the prenatal maturation of the immune system is expendable. Indeed, a majority of these immune maturation events will never be repeated once their prenatal "window" has passed. Seeding of the brain, lung and skin with macrophages, selection of useful T cells in the thymus, and formation of the gut's own mini-immune system are fundamental processes your baby needs as the foundation for a lifetime of good health. Protecting the developing immune system from insult is simple and effective. The alternative is a higher risk of immune-based diseases that require a lifetime of medical care.

Now that you have a general idea of immune maturation, including the ways in which immune cells spread throughout the entire body, we will turn our attention to a more overall view of the child's immune system. In the next three chapters we will look at how the pregnancy itself affects the development of the immune system, and we will compare the features of a healthy immune system with those of a dysfunctional immune system.

Overview of the Developing Immune System

- Development of the immune system occurs largely during gestation but some important steps happen after birth.
- Many one-time maturation steps happen during immune development that are never repeated in later life.

- Disruption of those one time events can cause immune damage that persists throughout life.
- These events help to define critical windows of immune vulnerability for your child.
- During these windows, extra care is needed for the long-term health of the immune system.

Chapter 6 — The Special Conditions of Pregnancy and the Immune System

Pregnancy Primer

In both biological and personal terms, one of the amazing life events is a successful pregnancy and the delivery of a healthy baby. The newborn baby has genetic material provided by both the mother and the father that comes in the form of DNA. The DNA is located primarily in chromosomes in the nucleus of cells but also in small structures called mitochondria (they are provided via the egg by the mother). The new baby combines features of the mother and father (e.g., the mother's eye color, the father's chin structure) and also has her or his own uniqueness. This results from the precise combinations of genes and their various forms (called alleles) that may never have occurred together in this pattern in any prior individual.

Most people are aware that pregnancy can be a challenging time for parents, particularly for the mother. Many physiological changes occur, and it is natural to focus on the visual, more obvious and frequently exciting changes associated with pregnancy. For example, the first ultrasound image of the baby or the feel of the baby's first movements usually produces a lot of excitement. But underneath, all of these changes that can be seen and felt, the immune system is also undergoing rapid change. Not only is the baby's immune system developing in the womb, the mother's immune system is also responding to her fetus. This chapter considers the impact of pregnancy and gestation on the immune systems of both the mother and the developing baby and why this is an important consideration in overall strategies to protect the baby's immune system.

Immune Protection Against Foreign Invasion of the Body

The immune system is designed, in part, to detect, remove and/or destroy foreign materials that invade the body including viruses, bacteria, parasites and also defective cells produced by the individual's own body, for example, tumor cells. To do this the immune system needs both an elaborate security system to warn of an intruder and the capability of forcibly removing the intruder before any harm is done. The first part of this security system is based on the identification of what are normal tissues and cells and what are foreign tissues or cells. The immune system's ability to discriminate between self cells and foreign cells is what makes organ transplants such a challenge. Usually, the transplanted organs have to be a close genetic match, and the recipient must receive immunosuppressive drug therapy for life. If the immune system is not sufficiently suppressed, the recipient's immune system will recognize the transplanted cells as foreign and will mount an attack that destroys the transplanted organ.

A Fetus Appears Foreign to the Mother's Immune System

What does a heart or kidney transplant have to do with pregnancy, you might ask? Recall that half of the chromosomes and DNA of the developing fetus come from the father. That means that the surfaces of the fetus' cells are coated with both the mother's and the father's proteins. The mother's immune system sees the father's proteins as foreign, and normally it would consider them to be a threat and ripe for destruction. Mother-father hybrid proteins also look foreign to the mother. So why is the half-foreign fetus not rejected by the mother like a transplanted heart or kidney would be without immunosuppressive drugs? Well, in rare cases this does appear to happen. Among women who have repeated miscarriages (more than three), there is evidence that the fetus may be seen as foreign by the mother and destroyed. But in the vast majority of pregnant women, the rejection response never happens. How is the mother's immune system tricked into tolerating the partially-foreign fetus and allowing it to grow and develop inside her?

Avoiding Immune Rejection of the Fetus — Immune Skewing

The placenta, the fetus and the mother's immune system use several tricks to avoid rejection and miscarriage. 1) Specialized immune cells (uterine natural killer cells and dendritic cells in the mucous membrane lining the uterus) surrounding the placenta help minimize problematic exposure of the mother's immune cells to the paternal proteins on the surfaces of fetal cells. 2) There are other cells (trophoblasts — cells that are part of the placenta) that try to send out signals that the fetus is privileged and should not be attacked. 3) The mother's normal immune function undergoes a shift, and for the majority of gestation, the mother's immune system suppresses the organ rejection part of its function. In fact, the entire prenatal environment is characterized by a targeted suppression of certain immune responses. There is a temporary skewing of immune function in both mother and child to protect the fetus. Evidence of immune system skewing comes from women who repeatedly miscarry. We now know many of them are not able to skew their immune systems enough to avoid the organ transplant type of response. Fortunately, some immune suppressing drug therapies can help these women to maintain a pregnancy to term.

Terminology of the Fetus-Protecting Immune Skewing

The type of immune skewing necessary to protect the fetus from maternal attack involves suppression of thymus-derived cells. Specifically, suppression targets Th1 cells and cytotoxic T lymphocytes: the immune cells that promote foreign tissue rejection. Because the mother's Th1 activity is temporarily reduced during pregnancy, the fetus remains unharmed. Other parts of the mother's immune system are not suppressed, and they may become predominant or appear to be relatively enhanced during pregnancy. Among these is immune system activity promoted by Th2 type cells. In general, pregnancy is considered to be dominated by Th2 activity, and this is particularly true of the middle and latter stages of the pregnancy. While a woman's normal immune balance has Th1 equal to Th2, during much of pregnancy Th2 is greater than Th1. The reduced Th1 function helps ensure that the woman's immune system will not reject the fetus.

How the Pregnancy Causes Immune Skewing

The changes in immune function within the pregnant woman are thought to be due at least in part to changes in the levels of sex hormones as well as pituitary and adrenal hormones. Among the hormones that can exert profound influences on the immune system are: estrogen, progesterone, prolactin, and various precursors and forms of testosterone. Many immune cells carry receptors for hormones and respond differently depending upon the concentrations of specific hormones. As discussed in a later chapter, the sensitivity of immune cells to endocrine changes is one of the reasons there is great concern over the level of endocrine-disrupting chemicals in our environment and the potential impact of these chemicals on health.

Impact of Pregnancy and Immune Skewing on the Mother

Obviously, the mother needs all of her immune functions, and it would not be healthy to lack Th1 function over the course of a lifetime. Fortunately, the pregnancy-timed depression in this immune function is of a short enough duration and a low enough level of reduction that the mother's health is rarely in jeopardy. However, the change can have certain noticeable effects. For example, the pregnant woman may experience an increase in the severity of certain immune or inflammatory-based diseases or a reduction in symptoms of others, depending upon which part of the immune system is involved in that specific disease. For example, the autoimmune disease rheumatoid arthritis is dependent more on Th1 function (Th1 function that has been misdirected against the body) than on Th2 function. Symptoms of this disease are reduced in a majority of pregnant women during much of pregnancy. However, the symptoms invariably return and increase dramatically after delivery during the post-partum period as the hormone balance changes again and Th1 immune function is restored to normal levels.

In contrast, a different autoimmune condition, systemic lupus erythematosus, also known as SLE or lupus, relies more on Th2 function than does rheumatoid arthritis to produce disease symptoms. In many pregnancies, women with this condition experience major flares of lupus, since pregnancy creates an environment where Th2 immune function is stronger. Pregnant women usually experience changes in the severity of allergic symptoms as well, although whether the symptoms are more or less severe depends both on the nature of the allergic conditions themselves (e.g., rhinitis, asthma, dermatitis or celiac) and on the timing of the pregnancy relative to the time of year and the possible seasonality of allergies. However, most women will note some change in the pattern of their allergy symptoms during pregnancy.

Impact of Pregnancy and Immunity Skewing on the Fetus

The special environment created in the mother to prevent her immune system from rejecting the developing fetus also has effects on the immune development of the fetus. Not surprisingly, the organ-rejection type of immune reactions that are prohibited in the mother during most of the pregnancy are also not allowed to develop fully in the fetus. As a result, the baby must catch up after birth. The Th2-predominant environment of the pregnant woman also characterizes the immune environment of the fetus. During normal pregnancies, the fetus' Th2 function develops rapidly while Th1 function is significantly delayed. It is important that this fetal immune imbalance not persist beyond birth.

The Baby Plays Immune Catch-Up Starting at Birth

At birth the baby's immune system has all the players needed for the full range of immune responses. However, the conditions imposed by the interaction between the fetus and the mother delay the development of the baby's cellular immune capabilities. The strategies to protect a child's immune system that are discussed in subsequent chapters have two important goals: 1) to protect the fetus from environmental factors and conditions that impair immune system development both prenatally and after birth, and 2) to promote neonatal conditions that help the newborn's immune capabilities reach their full capacity. It is important for parents to realize that no strategy covering both prenatal and childhood periods would be complete without both protection against harmful immune effects and promotion of healthy immune maturation. In fact the catch-up starts at birth. In recent years how the baby is born (Caesarian vs. vaginal delivery) has been shown to influence the maturation of the newborn's immune system. The most recent research indicates that vaginal delivery appears to give the developing immune system a useful boost toward maturity.

Overview of Pregnancy and Immunity

- Because the fetus makes proteins derived from the father's genes, it is partly foreign to the mother's immune system.
- Under normal circumstances, the mother's immune system would attack the fetus because of these foreign proteins from the father's genes.
- Special protections help maintain the pregnancy:
  - — 1) both the mother's and fetus' immune systems are skewed
  - — 2) maturation of part of the baby's immune system is delayed.
- Immune skewing and delayed maturity must be corrected at birth for the newborn to fight diseases effectively.
- Environmental factors can interfere with the corrections to the immune system that are needed for it to mature properly.

Chapter 7 — The Healthy Immune System at Work

Introduction

Previous chapters described the basic features of the immune system, how the immune system develops and how pregnancy affects the course of immune development. In order to illustrate the problems that can occur when childhood immune dysfunction occurs, we will first consider what the healthy immune system looks like in a child. In this chapter, we will describe some primary characteristics of an effective immune system: one that is in good balance, one that is firing on all cylinders, but one that is not out of control.

For an individual child, genetic background can influence exactly what immune balance can be obtained, and this is not the same for everyone. Individual differences notwithstanding, the vast majority of children without immune damage have the ability to fight off viruses, bacteria, parasites, fungal infections and tumor cells without attacking their own tissues and organs. The immune system knows when to use a particular type of response for maximum effectiveness and when a response is no longer needed and should be shut off. It knows how to combine short-term innate immunity and longer-term, specific acquired immunity for maximum effectiveness. It means that the immune system knows when its destructive forces are needed and when the process of healing diseased tissue should be started.

Because of genetic differences, not every child will have a perfectly balanced immune system. But it is possible to help our children avoid developmental hazards to their immune system and give them the best chance for a healthy life. We will now take a closer look at what a healthy immune system can accomplish on a daily basis.

Innate and Acquired Immunity Working Together in Your Child

In a healthy immune system, the two previously mentioned branches of immune function collaborate to provide protection. Innate immunity has several cellular players: natural killer cells, macrophages and neutrophils are the principle cells. They respond quickly to infection or tumor challenge, recognize specific molecules on the surfaces of pathogens or infected cells, and can kill microbes in a matter of minutes to hours. They do not need to divide and produce any daughter cells, which in the language of immunology means they don't need to be cloned. Innate immunity is influenced by the activity of other immune cells such as mast cells, lymphocytes, dendritic cells and basophils. Because innate immunity is less specific than acquired immunity, surrounding tissues may be damaged as well. We often call this inflammation. The immune system does not "remember" that the reason it started an innate immune response was to defend against an invading microbe, and its activities can spill over onto the body's own cells, harming them with "friendly fire." As far as the innate immune response is concerned, each infection is completely new as has never been seen before.

In contrast, acquired immunity is highly specific. It is directed against molecules on the surfaces of microbial pathogens and tumor cells, and it involves mainly lymphocytes (T and B cells), which are helped by dendritic cells and macrophages. Lymphocytes carry receptors on their surfaces that recognize the antigenic molecules on the invaders. Their recognition stimulates them to divide over and over again creating thousands of daughter cells (aka. clones) to go into battle. The cloning of B and T cells takes several days to weeks. Thus, acquired immunity is a strong and specific defensive force, but it is slow. If we only had acquired immunity and lacked innate immunity, most of us would die young due to rapidly spreading infections outrunning the cloning of our lymphocytes. On the other hand, acquired immunity usually does less collateral damage to tissues than innate immunity. A further advantage of acquired immunity is that the second time the same virus shows up, the response is quicker and much stronger than the first time. That is why many vaccination protocols use booster shots. The "memory" of the first vaccination makes the second response to the virus stronger, more specific and longer-lived. Some acquired immune responses protect us for decades.

We need acquired immunity to provide enough protection to defeat pathogens. Innate immunity alone is not enough for the huge number of pathogens a child will face. Your child needs both arms of immune defense.

Protecting the Doorways or "Avenues" of Infection and Toxic Exposure

The locations where the immune system first encounters an invading virus, bacterium, parasite, fungal spore or foreign object are the mouth, G.I. tract, skin, eyes, airways and urogenital tract. When contact occurs, macrophage-like cells (including dendritic cells) act as sentry cells and have three responsibilities: 1) detect the pathogen and recognize it as foreign, 2) engulf and remove the pathogen from the body, destroy it on-site or wall it off as a last resort, and 3) recruit other immune cells to fight that specific pathogen as needed. The first two steps in this defense are inherent to these sentry cells. They happen each and every day in a child's life, and we are not even aware of it. Immune cells are able to destroy pathogens and stop an infection before it gets started. Even in the case of the splinter in Sara's finger, the immune cells will (1) detect it, (2) wall it off, (3) keep infection from starting around it and (4) help to move it to the skin's surface (where a parent with a pair of tweezers can finish the job).

If step three is needed, the sentry cells recruit other immune cells to help. These may include neutrophils, natural killer cells, lymphocytes, basophils, eosinophils or mast cells depending upon the type of infectious agent. With the exception of lymphocytes, these cells usually go to the invader's location. Most lymphocytes, on the other hand, require that pathogen-containing dendritic cells come to them in the lymph nodes first. If this is a second visit to the child by the pathogen, the lymphocytes are ready to rush to the site of infection on short notice.

In a healthy immune system, the child has flexibility as to the numbers and kinds of immune cells that get involved. It is a matter of calling up the most qualified immune cells held in reserve that are best suited to the task and only as many as are needed at that time. Some of this mobilization is quick for calling in cells like natural killer cells and neutrophils. At first infection, lymphocytes will take longer. Ideally, the initial invasion is contained near the site where the pathogen enters, and none of the child's tissues are significantly affected.

When this works well, the virus your child breathed in at school, the bacteria that entered the barely visible scrape your child got on the playground and the small amount of bacteria present in the apple that was dropped on the ground before being eaten are all killed with little notice, discomfort or inconvenience. That is a healthy and effective immune surveillance system at work. As was discussed in Chapter 4 "Introduction to the Immune System," different types of immune responses are needed to combat different types of infections (viral, bacterial, parasitic, fungal) and tumors.

Immunological Memory

One of the novel features of the mature immune system is its capacity to know if it has ever seen a specific pathogen before. This is called "immunological memory." Very long-lived T and B lymphocytes provide this function. Because of immunological memory, the immune system is able to mount a very fast, intense and focused response against a pathogen that it is seeing for the second time. As previously mentioned, immunological memory is the basis of vaccination programs against pathogens. Memory responses can provide decades of protection.

A full capacity for immunological memory requires prenatal immune development as well as unimpeded maturation of the immune system after birth. In fact, it is the newborn and infancy periods when immune memory really starts to take off. So it would be erroneous to assume that once the baby is born, immune development is totally complete, and we no longer need to worry about toxins disrupting its ability to mature.

Organ and Tissue Maintenance

Immune cells reside in most tissues and organs of the body. This includes many locations that are rarely thought of as being associated with the immune system (e.g., testes, brain, liver). When the immune system is working effectively, immune cells collaborate with tissue cells in a beautiful synergy of functions.

Within organs, the specialized cells of the organ (e.g., hepatocytes in the liver, beta cells in the pancreas, myocytes in the heart) perform their functions, and the immune cells (like resident macrophages) in the same organ adapt their morphology and specific activity to fit the "style" of their new home. In turn, the immune cells constantly sample the environment, alert the organ to danger, provide defense against attack, take out the trash (remove dead and dying cells) and help with repairs. But the immune cells also influence the activity level of the non-immune cells in the organ and can impact the overall well-being of the organ. For this reason, we want the resident immune cells to function in a measured way in our organs to avoid both misdirected and excessive reactions. There is little room for collateral damage in a child where organs like the brain or heart are concerned. With a well-balanced and healthy immune system, the chances of immune-inflicted tissue damage can be minimized.

Conclusions

A well-functioning immune system provides the child with an important foundation for a long, healthy life. During the course of a lifetime, the child will face many different types of disease challenges. These will need to be met by the full range of immune functions. But the child's immune response must: 1) be specific for the challenge at hand (e.g., viral, bacterial, parasitic or fungal infection), 2) be measured so it meets the level of the threat without overdoing it, and 3) persist only as long as it is needed to protect health.

The template for immune balance and effective immune function is set early in life. This template can dramatically influence the risk of diseases during every decade of a child's life. This chapter has described why, when and where many different kinds of immune responses are needed for good health. The next chapter will provide examples of what can happen when this all goes very wrong. There are forks in the road to be taken during the critical windows of immune development and avoiding the pitfalls of immune damaging environmental conditions is an important first step. We can help the child head down a path toward more effective immunity over his/her lifespan and give him/her the opportunity to hold a great grandchild.

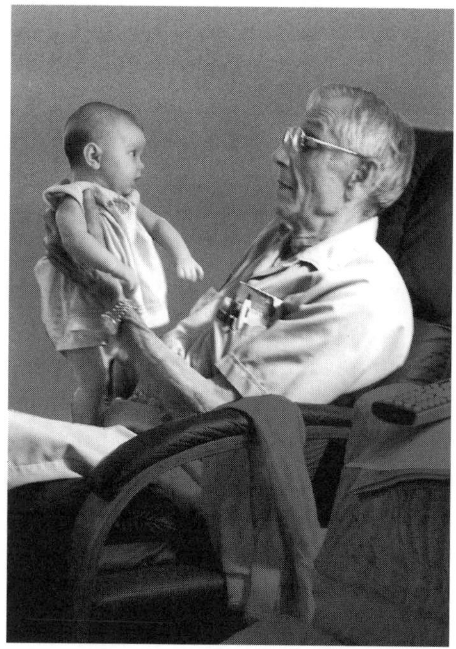

Overview of the Healthy Immune System

- A healthy immune system is able to fight viruses, bacteria, parasites and tumor cells with equal efficiency.
- It knows when to start fighting and when the battle is won.
- It minimizes collateral damage and avoids friendly fire.
- It balances use of innate and acquired immunity.
- It balances Th1 and Th2 responses.
- It is only moderately sensitive to stress.
- It avoids being tricked into attacking itself (autoimmunity) or into unhelpful responses against innocuous substances (allergy).

Chapter 8 — The Dysfunctional Immune System and Its Features

Introduction

The previous chapter described the features of a healthy, well-functioning immune system. When the immune system is in a healthy balance, a full range of appropriate immune responses are available to the child for defense against the variety of pathogens out there. The child's immune system is also able to discern between which cells belong to the child's body and which cells are foreign invaders. Plus, the immune system avoids allergic responses directed against harmless substances.

Not every child can have a perfect immune system. A small percentage of children will be genetically predisposed for immune system imbalances, regardless of whether they experienced problematic environmental exposures. But for the vast majority of children, their immune systems can perform just fine as long as the children are kept out of harm's way, and their immune systems are allowed to develop without significant insult. Understanding what a damaged immune system might look like, knowing what environmental conditions may be harmful for the developing immune system and understanding how better to protect our children represents a good portion of the rest of this book.

This chapter introduces immune dysfunction as both a major concern for children's health and an underlying basis for a lifetime of chronic diseases. In this chapter we describe why the prenatal, infancy and childhood periods deserve extra attention and extra protection. These are the most sensitive "windows" for an environmental damage to the immune system that results in persistent immune dysfunction. In fact, research indicates that these periods are particularly vulnerable to environmental impact. Worse, those periods are exquisitely important for later life immune function. Because of these facts, we wrote this book to help inform parents and their doctors. With better protection of the developing immune system, the child should have a much better chance of avoiding immune-based diseases.

It would take a whole book by itself to present detailed descriptions of all the possible combinations of environmentally-induced immune dysfunctions that have been observed. That is not the purpose of the present book. Instead, we will describe five of the more common examples that have been seen both in humans and with experimental research. Amongst these examples it will be obvious that developmental immunotoxicity (DIT) can result in several different patterns of immune dysfunction, and increased health risks are a result of the immune problems. In fact, more often than not, a given pattern of immune dysfunction will impact more than one category of diseases (infectious diseases, cancer, autoimmune diseases, allergic diseases, inflammatory diseases). The patterns of diseases associated with dysfunctional immune patterns are discussed in more detail in Chapter 11 "The Disease Progression Matrix."

The lessons we have learned in examining environmental impact on the developing immune system are that when things go wrong with the developing immune system, they can go very wrong and can last for a very long time. Hopefully, the cases described later in this chapter will serve as a reminder to parents and physicians to examine situations where immune dysfunction may play a role in current or future health risks. The cases illustrated in this chapter mention only a few of the environmental factors and conditions that can negatively affect the child's immune system. A more complete discussion of the various environmental risk factors is presented in later chapters of the book.

The Targets of Environmentally-Induced Immune Dysfunction

Virtually all of the components of the immune system that were discussed in the prior chapters have been described as targets of early-life environmental exposures and conditions. Targets range from the thymocytes in the prenatal thymus to brain and lung macrophages, mast cells, neutrophils, antibody-producing B lymphocytes, dendritic cells, basophils, eosinophils, intraepithelial lymphocytes, and the entire spectrum of T lymphocytes that regulate immune responses (Tregs, Th1, Th2, and Th17 cells). The development, differentiation and function of the cell populations can be affected in different combinations by toxins that produce different patterns of immune dysfunction and associated disease risk in the child.

Critical Windows of Immune Vulnerability

Chapter 5 described how the immune system develops. Of note is the fact that prenatal and infant development can be divided into a series of defined steps or windows for the immune system. When the window represents a one-time-only immune maturation event, or it is a necessary building-block for later immune maturation, it is called a "critical window." Critical windows of immune vulnerability were first described in a 2000 workshop publication and were later updated in 2006 as more DIT data became available. Examples of critical windows of immune vulnerability are shown in Figure 8.1. Specific toxic chemicals or drugs have been reported to disrupt each of these windows.

Figures 8.1a and 8.1b show that different chemicals and drugs can disrupt the developing immune system at specific critical windows during stages of fetal development. These disruptions result in a dysfunctional immune system and increase the risk of specific diseases.

The immune events that occur during these critical developmental windows are the building blocks for the later immune system. One maturational event is stacked on top of another in sequence. Everything the immune system will be asked to do in the child is largely based on having this sequence of immune maturation events occur both successfully and without delay. For most of the developmental events in the immune system, there is no do-over.

What happens during each critical window of development for the immune system is usually a distinct and active process (e.g., cells move, cells die, cells change) that, when combined, help the immune system get everything into place for adequate protection of the child. There is no step in this maturation process that is expendable when it comes to good health. A missed step during the selection process of T lymphocytes in the thymus can dramatically increase the risk of both immunosuppression and

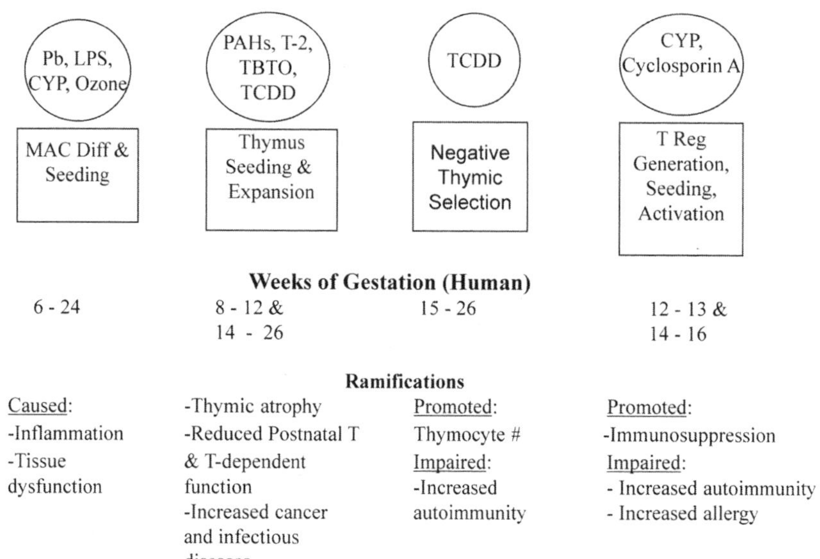

Figure 8.1a. Critical windows for DIT. Pb = Lead, LPS = bacterial endotoxin, CYP = cyclophosphomide, PAHs = polycyclic aromatic hydrocarbons, T-2 = an agricultural fungal toxin, TBTO = tributyltin, TCDD = a dioxin, cyclosporin A = an immunosuppressant drug used in organ transplants.

autoimmunity. Likewise, improper maturation of macrophages in the third trimester can have an immediate effect on the infant's resistance to bacteria and on the risk of inflammatory disease as the child ages. Impaired dendritic cell maturation can affect childhood resistance to viruses, and improper seeding of immune cells to the brain and G.I. tract is a concern for later disease involving these tissues.

In the next section, we describe some prominent patterns of immune dysfunction that are seen in early life and that affect the risk of chronic disease both during childhood and in the adult.

Prominent Patterns of a Dysfunctional Immune System in Children

Example 1 — Reduced Defense Against Infectious Diseases

Researchers from Harvard University and Denmark found that when pregnant women ate high polychlorinated biphenyl (PCB; detailed in

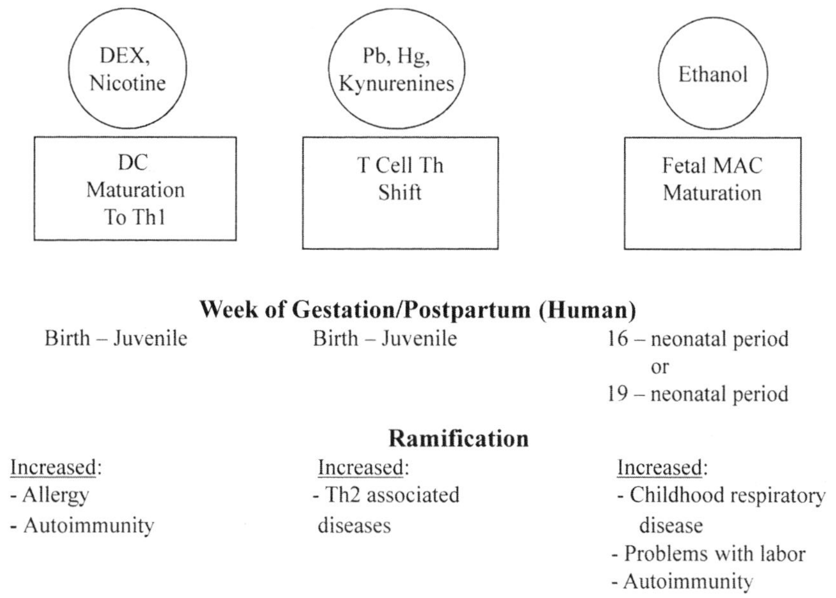

Figure 8.1b. Critical windows for DIT. DEX = Dexamethasone, Pb = lead, Hg = mercury, kynurenines = a body metabolite, ethanol = an alcohol.

Chapter 16)-contaminated seafood, their children had an inadequate response to childhood vaccinations. They were able to determine this by measuring the level of PCBs in the cord blood after the baby's birth.

PCB intake in early life was also shown to be related to the risk of recurrent ear infections in several populations of children in both North America and Europe (where there was a high seafood diet). The combination of the reduced response to childhood vaccines and the increased incidence of childhood infections describes one dysfunctional pattern where environmental exposures produce gaps in the immune system's ability to respond to certain infectious diseases. PCBs are not the only toxin capable of producing immunosuppression following in utero exposure.

Example 2 — Allergy and Autoimmunity Occurring Together

Evidence from both human studies and experimental research suggests that exposure to heavy metals such as lead and mercury (see Chapter 16) can produce several changes to the developing immune system that result in dysfunction. Several of the heavy metals can act on dendritic cells causing them to favor fetal-like Th2 responses over Th1 responses. Of course, this has the possibility of reducing some cell-mediated immune responses that are needed for protection against infections and cancer. What heavy metals definitely do is increase the risk of IgE production and thus increase the risk of allergic disease.

Depending upon the amount of heavy metal contained in the exposure and the timing of when it occurs in early life, the pattern of T lymphocyte development is also disrupted. This disruption appears to increase the risk of some Th2-dependent autoimmune diseases such as lupus. While lupus may show up much later in life than childhood allergies, the pattern for higher risk of autoimmunity is already set by birth or in infancy. This combination of greater risk of allergies and later life lupus is one that is seen with developmental immunotoxicity (DIT).

Example 3 — Immunosuppression, Inflammation and Autoimmunity All Together

Dioxin (the most common form of which is also known as 2,3,7,8-tetrachlorodibenzo-p-dioxin, TCDD; see Chapter 16) is one of the more potent early-life immune and reproductive toxins. Exposure of the developing immune system to TCDD appears to cause a pattern of immune disruption that focuses on the thymus and developing T cells. But the impact of the disruption also affects several other immune cell populations in the offspring. Exposure to TCDD produces focused immunosuppression that makes the baby more susceptible to some infectious diseases. However, along with this researchers have found that in some situations, inflammatory responses are out of control, and the increased inflammation damages tissues that lead to additional disease concerns.

If immunosuppression and damaging inflammation are not enough, the impact of TCDD exposure does not end there. Even with the focused immunosuppression and potential for inflammation-inflicted tissue damage, there is also disrupted use of receptors on T cells and reduced Treg function that increases the risk of autoimmune disease. Not all of these immunotoxic outcomes will necessarily be apparent until they are triggered by something (infection, second toxic exposure, stress, trauma) at a later date. But the pattern of a combination of some suppressed immune responses, some inappropriate inflammation and a higher chance of autoimmunity becomes established by early-life exposure to TCDD.

This example with TCDD illustrates that several different problems can arise for the developing immune system from exposure to just one environmental factor.

Example 4 — Allergy, Infection, Inflammation and Increased Cancer Risk Together

Cigarette smoke is one of the environmental pollutants of greatest concern for the child's immune system (see Chapter 16). It is also one of the developmental immunotoxicants that is the easiest to control. Early exposure to cigarette smoke produces a complex pattern of immune dysfunction that includes virtually every category of immune dysfunction and health concern known. Perhaps that is not completely surprising since cigarette smoke contains many different individual chemicals that are potent toxins.

It is clear that early-life exposure to cigarette smoke alters both dendritic cell and macrophage activities and the host defenses in the lung. Risk of respiratory allergies including childhood asthma and wheezing is increased as is the susceptibility to certain respiratory infections. Oxidative damage of the lung is greater in infants from mothers who smoked during pregnancy. This suggests that a greater chance of inflammatory damage exists in those children. The increased inflammatory damage can result from increased oxygen radical production, reduced antioxidant activity in tissues or both of these in combination.

Research evidence also suggests that cell-mediated immunity against tumors is decreased in offspring that were exposed to cigarette smoke. Therefore, their overall risk of cancer may be greater. The disruption of innate immune maturation in the lungs and in antigen presentation by dendritic cells has consequences that affect the risk of several different categories of diseases. Again, some of these like allergies and asthma, increased infections and increased inflammation are likely to show up in the child. However, the higher risk of cancer may not become apparent until later in life (i.e., adulthood).

Example 5 — Inflammation, Depression and Metabolic Problems Together

Excessive inflammation produced by the dysfunctional immune system, clinical depression and even occasionally metabolic problems seem to go hand-in-hand. This reflects the close communication and interactions between the immune, neurological and endocrine systems. Dysfunction in any one of these systems can have significant ramifications for the others. In some publications, this is referred to as "inflamm-aging." The reason is that prolonged even low level inflammation throughout childhood and in the young adult is associated with a significant number of diseases of later life. These include both atherosclerosis as well as Alzheimer's disease.

Numerous environmental factors, including what pregnant women eat and drink, are capable of disrupting the developing immune system in a way that leads to inappropriate and/or excessive inflammation in the child. For example, in utero exposure to arsenic appears to produce this pattern of immune dysfunction. In several settings this dysfunctional inflammation is associated with an increased likelihood of one or more of the following: depression, metabolic problems (obesity and metabolic syndrome) and cardiovascular disease. This "pattern" is known to be readily established in early life. One of the hallmarks of the Example #5 immune dysfunctional pattern is the overproduction of the cytokines, TNF-alpha and IL-6, both of which are associated with inflammation.

Conclusions

Prenatal and childhood-induced immune dysfunction can come in an almost unlimited number of combinations or patterns. In fact, it now appears that having only immunosuppression or allergy (a form of hypersensitivity) or improper inflammation alone is rarer than having some combination of immune problems as a result of early-life environmental insult. In this chapter we have introduced five common and significant patterns of immune dysfunction that follow an in utero exposure to toxic chemicals. It is clear that any one of these patterns is associated with an increased risk of several diseases. Both the environmental factors and conditions producing these patterns and the diseases that result from them are discussed in more detail in subsequent chapters of this book.

Overview of the Dysfunctional Immune System

- It comes in many different permutations and forms.
- Responses may be too little, too late or the wrong kind .
- Responses may not shut off well and can cause tissue damage or exhaust the immune system.
- It may be tricked into autoimmune or allergic responses.
- It may be overly sensitive to stress.
- It may have skewed T helper function favoring Thl or Th2.
- It may have inadequate or inappropriate innate immune responses.
- It may have undisciplined inflammatory responses.
- Any combination of the above is possible.

Chapter 9 — Avenues for Immune Exposure

Introduction

Our bodies are exposed to the environment in a variety of ways such as through the air we breathe, the food we eat, the water we drink and the surfaces we touch or that touch us. Fortunately, our airways, gastrointestinal tract, skin and eyes have purposely designed barriers to help protect us against harmful interactions. Nasal hairs help filter out large particles and bacteria in the air. Our gastrointestinal tract comes equipped with acids to digest or kill many things that could cause us harm and the capacity to expel other contents that are upsetting to our stomachs. Our skin allows small molecules in but is also a barrier against invasion by bacteria that surround us. Our eyes have specialized antibody-containing secretions better known as tears. These help to protect against pollutants and pathogens. It is easy for us to take for granted just how these protective barriers help our children. But they are very important as a front line of defense.

What happens when chemicals, drugs, pathogens or physical agents make it past these barriers? It should come as no surprise that one of the first things that harmful substances and agents encounter are immune cells. As previously mentioned, immune cells can be found in virtually every tissue and organ of the body. But the portals of exposure to the external environment (airways, gut, skin, eyes) not only have lots of immune cells present, they also have specialized forms of many immune cells. For example, alveolar macrophages in the lung are not really like other macrophages found elsewhere in the body. It is almost like they are from a different planet as macrophages go. The intraepithelial lymphocytes (IELs) of the gut are also a virtually unique population of lymphocytes with highly specialized features. The regions around the eye are rich in lymphocytes designed to produce IgA, which is an antibody that works best in secretions such as tears. The skin has types of specialized cells called Langerhans cells and keratinocytes. The former can act a little like dendritic cells in collecting antigens, travelling to the lymph node and presenting the antigens to T lymphocytes. Keratinocytes are epithelial-type cells present in the epidermal layer of skin. They act as an important barrier to toxins.

Every portal where the inside of our body can encounter the environment is rich in immune cells, and each portal has its own unique mix of immune cells with the best function to protect us at that site. But it also means that these populations of immune cells have their own vulnerabilities particularly in the young.

Children have basic differences in anatomy and metabolism from adults, and these differences predispose children to greater risk from environmental exposures. To sustain their smaller often more active bodies, children breathe more, eat differently and have more contact with more contaminated surfaces during play when compared with adults. The combination of increased exposure to environmental pollutants and an immune system that is less prepared to deal with toxins is why our children need special safety consideration and extra care to keep them out of harm's way.

This chapter will consider how environmental exposures through different portals may cause different challenges for the child's immune system.

The Airways

The airway system or respiratory tract includes the nose, sinuses, trachea and lungs. Exposure to air pollutants is a very serious issue for children. Part of this is based on some basic structural differences between children and adults. The lungs of children are smaller and their airways are narrower than those of adults. But children still must provide oxygen to their tissues for survival and growth. To get enough oxygen from their smaller lungs to the tissues, children need to breathe more often. The breathing rate, which is measured as breaths taken each minute, across all ages of children is higher than that of healthy adults. Young children are taking two breaths for every one taken by a normal adult. And that is if the child is resting rather than crawling, running, climbing or actively playing. In fact, the difference is so great that, even after strenuous exercise, an adult has a breathing rate barely reaching that of a resting preschool child. Even an adult's respiratory rate while jogging is lower than that of most infants.

What this means is that each minute children are likely to breathe in more of the toxins and allergens found in air than adults. The volume of air they inhale per pound of body weight is greater than that of their parents. By taking in that larger volume, they breathe in a greater amount of particles and toxic chemicals than the parent. So if a parent is carrying an infant through an area with high traffic pollution or visits a house with tobacco smokers for the day, the child is likely to take more pollutant particles into his or her lungs than the parent.

Even the reduced height of a child vs. that of a parent can mean that the child may have to deal with a higher level of exposure from airborne particles. Heavier particles in air are drawn down by gravity and tend to accumulate closer to the ground. This is the space where a child is sitting in a stroller, crawling or playing on the ground. So put a parent and a child in the same outdoor or indoor environment, and air pollutant exposure of the lungs is greater for the child. The greater exposure risk does not even consider whether the child's immune system in the lungs is ready to deal with all of these inhaled particles and toxic chemicals.

As will be discussed later with the skin, the airways have specific barriers to aide in the protection against pathogens and other unwelcome environmental insults. The respiratory tract has some normal microbial flora that can help to keep invading pathogens from establishing themselves. In our nasal secretions there are enzymes that can help to kill pathogens. Finally, the action of cilia in the respiratory tract, the flow of mucus and the airflow in general can all act to keep pathogens and toxic particles from reaching our lungs.

In Chapter 4 some of the specialized immune tissues of the airways were mentioned. These included the bronchus-associated lymphoid tissues (BALT), which is a collection of lymphocytes, dendritic cells and macrophages along the epithelial lining of the respiratory tract. In general the BALT is less well organized than the equivalent tissue in the G.I. tract (gastrointestinal lymphoid tissue, GALT). However, the presence of the BALT suggests that all components of the immune system in the airways are in place to respond in both protective and sometimes harmful ways following a challenge.

Among the specialized immune cells in the airways are alveolar macrophages. Unlike most other macrophages, alveolar macrophages are constantly exposed to the external environment. Their job is to collect dust and other particles we breathe in and destroy or remove them from our airways. That can be a problem when they encounter something that either impairs their function or that they cannot digest or remove. In fact, in some instances, the inability of macrophages to digest particles or fibers can be devastating for our lungs.

Both silica dust and asbestos are impossible for macrophages to digest. The result is usually lung damage and replacement with non-functioning material (lung fibrosis) or lung cancer. Other toxins produce more subtle problems for alveolar macrophages. Ozone, cigarette smoke, traffic pollutants, heavy metals and toxic gases in the air can either reduce the effectiveness of these cells in screening out and clearing bacteria, or they can cause the immune cells to indiscriminately damage the lung. Young children are a particularly vulnerable population, and when their lung tissue is damaged, it is difficult to fully restore its appropriate function. As a result, alveolar macrophages are a major target for protection of our children.

The G.I. Tract

The G.I. tract includes the mouth, esophagus, stomach and intestines. It represents the primary route of oral exposure to toxins, drugs and microbes. In children, oral exposure concerns go beyond just food and water. The normal activity of children can involve playing in soil, lawns or on other surfaces. Normal hand-to-mouth activity of young children means if they touch it, it also goes into their mouth. So some toxin and microbial exposures that would mainly involve only the skin in adults become significant oral exposures in children.

The immune cells in the G.I. tract extend protection throughout the entire system. For example, dendritic cells, macrophages and T lymphocytes guard our taste center. Since infections and inflammation can impair our sense of taste, the status of these immune cell populations is significant for nutrition-related quality of life. The salivary glands are on the frontline of oral immune protection. But other areas such as the tongue, adenoids and tonsils form an additional ring of immune protection around the oral cavity. The flow of fluid, mucous, food, saliva and the presence of stomach acid all help to reduce the chances that pathogens will take up residence in our G.I. tract.

In the lower areas of our G.I. tract, only a thin layer of epithelial cells separates our mucosal immune system from the gut flora (our digestive bacteria). That epithelial barrier's function is important, and it can be aided by some supplements such as probiotic bacteria. But there is an important difference between our skin barrier and its immune tissue and the tissues in our gut. The skin is essentially a barrier against all external microbes. But our gut epithelial lining contains specialized cells called microfold cells or "M" cells. They constantly sample the bacterial content of our gut and funnel that information to our G.I. tract immune cells.

We need our gut immune cells not only to become friends with good bacteria but to protect us from harmful bacteria. We also need the gut bacteria to stay in the proper place in the G.I. tract. Even usually harmless bacteria can be a problem when the mucosal immune barriers are broken and our normally friendly bacteria go places where they do not belong.

After the gut is injured by toxins, friendly bacteria send chemical signals to the T cells causing them to make antibacterial products, which help keep harmful bacteria from setting up shop in the injured gut. In the meantime, the T cells help the gut to repair itself. Once the gut is repaired and the hole in the lining is sealed, the immediate danger is over. If the friendly bacteria are too low in number or absent altogether, the T cells have problems repairing the gut, and the chance for harmful bacteria to start an infection is greater.

Children taking a course of antibiotics have their normal gut bacteria destroyed along with the harmful bacteria. Among these are gut-friendly *E. coli* that are able to: 1) block the areas on the gut lining where disease-causing bacteria could lodge and 2) secrete protective substances that help keep out harmful bacteria such as Salmonella. This means harmful bacteria may be able to get a foothold after the antibiotic treatment is completed at a time when the friendly gut bacteria are significantly lower in number. Additionally, the IELs will not function properly if there are not enough friendly gut bacteria. This interaction of G.I. tract immune cells and friendly bacteria is critical. When missing, it further increases the chance that another opportunistic pathogen will settle into the gut (e.g., Clostridium strains).

All of the G.I. tract immune cells are ready to respond to foreign antigens once the antigens are funneled through M cells or dendritic cells. The problem arises when the delicate balance of homeostasis, immune maintenance and protection in the gut goes wrong. Then inflammation, food allergies, nutrient malabsorption and disease are likely results. Keeping a good level of gut bacteria in place helps to prevent G.I. tract infections and inflammation plus food allergies.

The Skin

Exposure to toxicants through the skin is particularly important in children. If you consider the area of skin that covers a child per pound of weight compared to the area of skin covering an adult, the child has more skin per unit of weight. Essentially, that means that if all else is equal for the same exposure to pollutants, the child is at a greater risk for absorbing toxins through their skin than is the adult.

But all may not be equal for actual exposure, either. As discussed in a recent World Health Organization report on children and exposure to environmental chemicals, the normal behavior of children can put them at greater risk of exposure to environmental contaminants. Children crawl, climb and roll around on a variety of surfaces to a far greater extent than most adults. Even the author did as a child (see photo).

If any of the surfaces are contaminated with hazardous chemicals or pathogens, their exposure is likely to be greater than that of adults. Simply put, they are more likely to have skin contact with dirt, turf and fabricated surfaces that may heighten their exposure to toxins, such as lead.

As mentioned in the introduction to this chapter, skin contains highly specialized cell types that are important in protecting the individual via

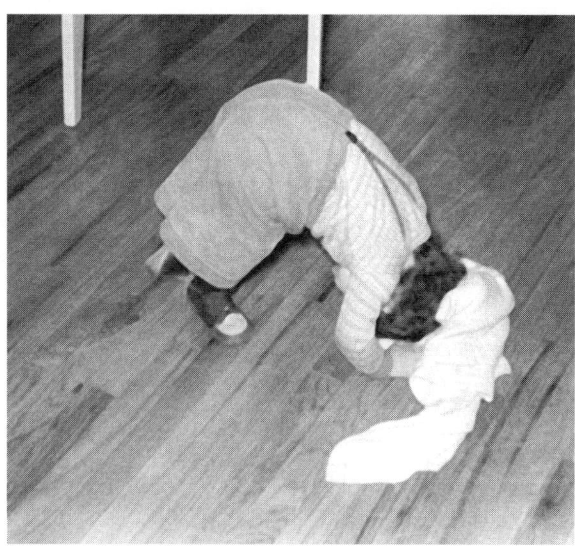

healthy immune responses. Langerhans cells are a relatively immature form of dendritic cells. These cells constantly collect antigens and display them to lymphocytes in the lymph nodes (regional receiving stations). Excessive ultraviolet radiation absorbed by the skin can alter Langerhans cell numbers or function and present a major health problem such as increased risk of infection or cancer.

Other specialized cells of the skin include the keratinocytes. These cells used to be thought of as a physical protective barrier in the epidermis. While they do serve that function, we now know they do much more. They have important immune functions. Keratinocytes can promote inflammation by producing certain by-products of metabolism. Plus, they can affect the direction of an immune response by producing cytokines such as IL-1, IL-3 and IL-6, which are involved in inflammatory immune responses. They can also help with the healing of wounds.

These cells are greatly influenced by the environment. We know that sunburn induced by ultraviolet light is largely a result of inflammation caused by keratinocytes in the skin. Ironically, there is some evidence that silver nitrate ointments used in burn patients slow, rather than speed up, the healing of the skin. This is because the metal causes the keratinocytes to die. Other metals such as arsenic also appear to have harmful effects on keratinocytes. Arsenic is a known skin carcinogen. But now it appears that part of the risk for arsenic-induced skin cancer is due to its harmful effects on the keratinocyte's ability to respond immunologically.

Even certain environmental insults that we would think of as being unrelated to the skin appear to affect the function of Langerhans cells and keratinocytes. For example, recent studies suggest that noise-induced stress increases the number of Langerhans cells in the skin, causes them to mature differently and causes keratinocytes to die. If allowed to continue, the noise-induced stress changes the numbers of cells present and their function in the skin. This in turn could promote an immune dermatitis-related disease.

The Eyes

The eyes represent an important portal to our environment. Like the skin, respiratory tract and G.I. tract, the eyes have natural defenses against pathogens and toxic exposure. The flow of tears serves to protect them against harmful exposures. Tears contain IgA antibodies and lysozymes, which are enzymes that can degrade and destroy bacteria.

The eye is also unique immunologically in what is called an "immune privileged site." This means that immune cells in the area tend to be naturally suppressed against reactions to components of the eye. Under normal circumstances, this helps to protect the internal portions of the eye from possible damage by the immune system.

Problems can occur if the eye is otherwise damaged and the dendritic cells then begin to see eye-associated antigens and present these to T lymphocytes. Normally, T lymphocytes will not have seen eye antigens before. So if the eye becomes damaged, T lymphocytes may think eye antigens are foreign and an autoimmune attack of the eye (called uvitis) can result. In fact, in children with other autoimmune and inflammatory conditions, such as juvenile rheumatoid arthritis, sarcoidosis and lupus, the eye can become involved as well.

Ironically, damage in one eye can lead to autoimmune reactions against the unaffected eye. For example, laser burn of the retina in one eye can cause a loss of immune privilege. The resulting immune response can involve the eye that was not damaged by the laser once the privilege is lost.

It is important to recognize that immune privilege of the eye itself does not stop eye allergy (also called allergic conjunctivitis) from happening. As with other immune responses, eye allergy is usually a Th2-driven response.

The eye is particularly sensitive to toxins as reflected by the number of household products that warn against eye irritation. Parents can aid the health of their child's eyes by recognizing that their eyes are a major portal to the environment. Not only can toxins enter the body through that route, but the risk of allergic eye disease and loss of immune privilege are significant health concerns. Protecting the eyes from damage can help to keep the immune system tolerant of the eye.

The Urogenital Tract

While the urogenital tract may appear to be of lesser concern as a route of immune exposure, particularly among children, it is not one to be totally ignored. Specialized immune cells such as testicular and ovarian macrophages reside in the reproductive organs. The health and well-being of these immune cells are important for the appropriate function of these organs in the adult. Urogenital infections and other exposures can affect the status of these immune cell populations. Like other regions exposed to the environment, the urogenital tract has some natural protection. Urine flow and the acidic environment of the urinary tract help to keep harmful bacteria from becoming established. While this portal can be affected by exposure to environmental toxins and drugs, less information is available about specific toxins and urogenital tract macrophages than for alveolar macrophages. Why protect the urogenital immune cells? It can pay dividends particularly later in life when prostate, bladder, kidney, testis and ovarian function can dramatically impact health and longevity.

Conclusions

The child has several major avenues or portals for immunological interaction with the environment. These include the airways, skin, gastrointestinal tract, eyes and urogenital tract. Not surprisingly these are possible routes of infection. But these avenues are also routes through which environmental toxins can readily invade and harm the immune cells. The immune damage can be either local to the site (e.g., lung) or throughout the body.

Additionally, the basic anatomy and physiology of the growing child causes the toxin exposure in these portal areas to be greater in children than adults. For this reason, environmental exposures that we might not think twice about as adults are magnified to a point of concern in children.

Overview of Avenues of Immune Exposure

- The airways, G.I. tract (mouth, stomach, intestines), skin and eyes are the main route for environmental exposure of immune cells.
- Specialized immune cells sit in each location (e.g., lungs, skin, eye) and would be exposed. But the effects may be either local or impact the entire immune system.
- Children may be exposed to a single chemical or drug via more than one avenue (e.g., metals in air, food/water or though contact with skin).

Chapter 10 — Diseases Stemming From Prenatal and Early Life Toxic Exposures

Introduction

Childhood illnesses are every parent's nightmare. We're all familiar with the late nights sitting beside a feverish child's bedside. Or the sniffling, sneezing and coughing that seems to haunt them every spring. Some illnesses seem fairly benign, like hayfever and skin rashes. And even asthma is often manageable with medications and inhalers. But some childhood illnesses can retard growth, as in pediatric celiac disease (the inability to tolerate gluten in grains), or delay neurological development as in autism and autism spectrum disorders. There are the ones that cause heart breaking pain like pediatric idiopathic arthritis. Then there are ones that are life-threatening — childhood leukemia and type 1 diabetes. What if there were common causal elements behind many of these? Some factors like genetics we have little control over and can merely hope for the best. But what if we could better control other factors that contribute to these illnesses? What if there were more we could do to reduce the risk of acquiring these illnesses and spare our children? Most of us are familiar with illnesses that are inherited, and many of us know some of the things that are in our homes and environment that can harm a child. But how many realize that early damage to the immune system can last a lifetime?

Let's take a look at the specific diseases that are influenced by the prenatal and infant environment and the health and well-being of the immune system. As a guide to these diseases, we have prepared two timelines of diseases with established or suspected immune involvement. The diseases on these timelines are varied, can produce a broad range of symptoms and may involve many different tissues and organs. The first timeline (Figure 10.1) shows the diseases and forms of diseases that generally

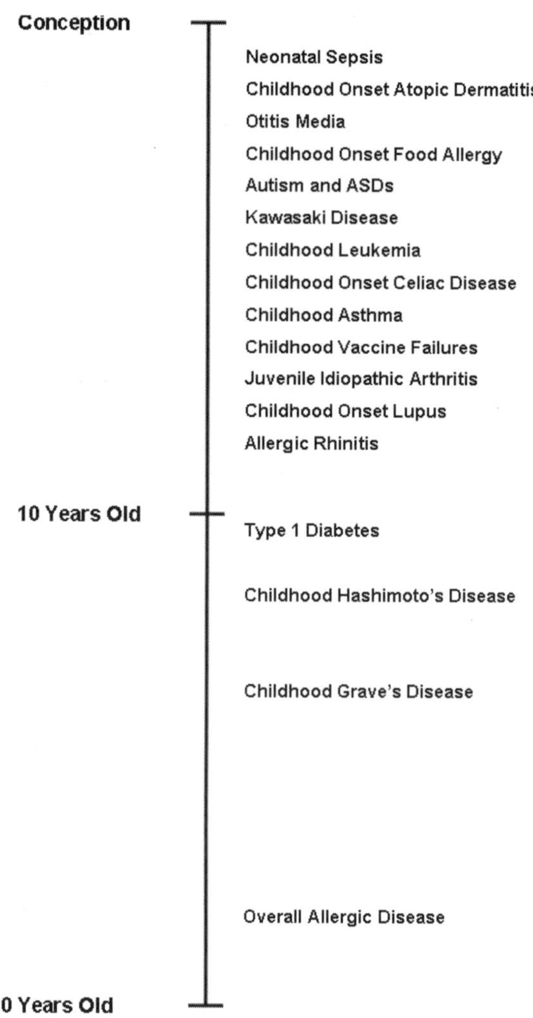

Figure 10.1. Immune-related diseases seen most in childhood with average ages of onset.

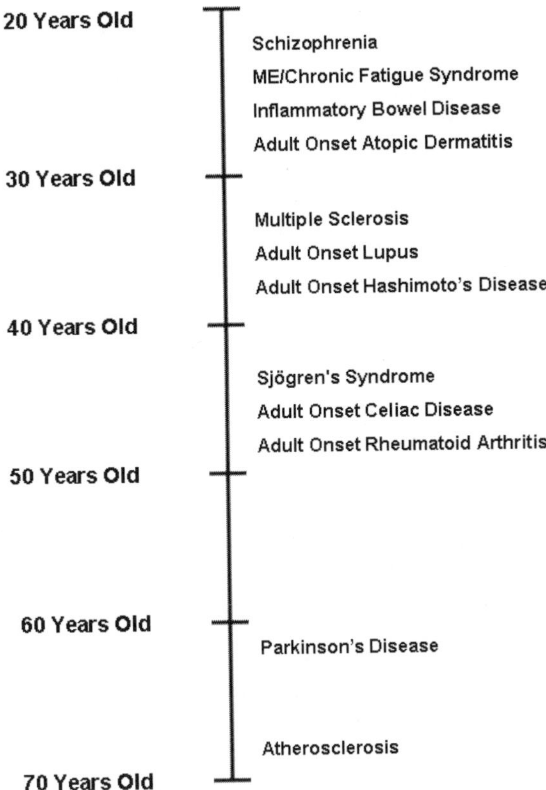

Figure 10.2. Immune-related diseases seen most in adults with average adult ages of onset.

appear between birth to 20 years of age (which for our purposes we are defining as childhood).

The second timeline (Figure 10.2) focuses on diseases usually seen between the ages of 20 and later life (adult). The placement of each disease along the childhood and adult timelines is meant to indicate the approximate average age when each disease appears. Many of these diseases can actually appear at any age, so the average age should just be used as a general guide.

Additionally, some of the diseases have been divided into childhood and adult forms. In some cases the childhood forms of the disease may present with a different range of symptoms or a different degree of severity from the adult-onset form of the disease. This is the case with childhood-onset vs. adult-onset celiac and lupus. The childhood form of each tends to be more severe and requires more intense therapy.

Taken together, these diseases represent a large percentage of all chronic diseases suffered by children. Most persist in the adult and will require lifelong medical treatment and therapy. These in turn have a negative impact on the child's quality of life and can present a serious economic burden on their families. Preventing or avoiding these diseases is a better option vs. life-long medication or therapy.

Allergic Disease and Asthma

Allergies, including asthma, are thought to affect between 15–25% of the population in most developed countries. Even a single allergic disease such as allergic rhinitis (hayfever) has been estimated to impact up to 20% of the U.S. population. While allergies can arise at any age, most first appear during childhood or at least by young adulthood and can worsen with age. The incidence of allergic disease has risen dramatically in developed nations in recent decades. Since our genetics do not change that rapidly, the increase is most likely due to environmental causes.

More recently, even developing countries have been reporting increases in asthma, atopic dermatitis (eczema) and allergic rhinitis. As chronic diseases, allergies and asthma usually affect the individual over the course of their entire life and may create difficult life changes such as getting rid of a beloved pet, restricting activity levels and/or negatively impacting activities during a particular period of the year (seasonal allergies). Allergies often require medical intervention in the form of prescription antihistamines, nasal steroid sprays, antihistamine and hydrocortisone creams, allergy shots, sublingual exposures or other approaches designed to alter the immune responses that are creating the symptoms. For less severe yet persistent allergic symptoms, individuals may spend decades purchasing over the counter allergy medications in an attempt to "live with" the condition.

Several allergic diseases have underlying immune dysfunction and environmental risks in common. For instance, if your newborn develops eczema, that child has over a 50% greater chance of developing another allergic condition, like allergic rhinitis, asthma or food allergies later in life. Several environmental, dietary and physical factors (such as abuse and low birth weight) have been reported to increase the risk of acquiring a childhood allergic disease. Other factors are thought to actually protect against these diseases. Most of the elements known or suspected to cause allergic diseases have one or more of four overlapping factors: (1) they cause the immune system to be skewed toward an overproduction of IgE, which is an allergy-promoting antibody, (2) they cause excessive and inappropriate inflammation in the airways, skin or gut, (3) they interfere with the regulatory network of lymphocytes and (4) they freeze some immune responses so the immune system acts more like that of a late fetus rather than that of a fully developed child.

Those environmental risk factors presently identified as contributing to childhood allergies cannot account for the prevalence and increase in the disease. There are obviously more problematic toxicants waiting to be identified. Risk factors during pregnancy and in the young child that are known or suspected to increase the risk of childhood allergies include: maternal smoking, passive or environmental tobacco smoke (often called ETS), maternal use of alcohol or recreational drugs and maternal acetaminophen (found in Tylenol, Excedrin and Midol) intake. Other factors include: intensive and early childhood vaccination protocols, side-effects of neonatal antibiotic use (which can be difficult to separate from the effects of the infections they are designed to treat), exposure to heavy metals (lead, cadmium, mercury), living near roads with heavy traffic, exposure to smoke from a wood stove, introduction of pets into a previously pet-free household in later childhood, specific dietary fat intake (levels and amounts of omega 6 vs. omega 3 dietary fatty acids), reduced levels of Vitamins E and D during pregnancy, Caesarian delivery vs. vaginal delivery, and specific respiratory infections in the young child (such as respiratory syncytial virus infection).

Thankfully, there are some factors that seem to reduce the risk of childhood allergies. Because a child's genetics also come into play, they cannot ensure that every child would be allergy-free if followed, but they are factors that can be controlled for a better outcome. These protective factors include: exposure to an environment with farm animals during pregnancy and during the early infant years, appropriate levels of

Vitamins E and D during pregnancy, some fatty fish in the diet (while avoiding as much mercury and PCBs as possible), having a pet in the household of a newborn, exposing the child to daycare earlier rather than later in life, delaying and/or separating some childhood vaccinations so young children don't receive such an intense grouping of live vaccines as early in life as has become the routine.

In fact, researchers at the University of Manitoba looked at the possible benefits of delaying childhood vaccinations. They studied 11,531 children, which is a significant population, in order to see what the effects would be of delaying vaccinations. They found that those children whose first dose of diphtheria-pertussis-tetanus (DPT) vaccine was delayed by at least two months had only half the rate of asthma by age seven than did those children who received the DPT vaccination at an earlier age. Although the researchers emphasized that additional validation studies are needed to support their findings, the results do seem to suggest that the trend toward moving childhood vaccinations to earlier and earlier ages presents a significant downside where immune-related diseases like allergies and asthma are concerned. The most likely explanation is that the younger child's immune system is not sufficiently mature to handle the vaccination in a balanced way.

Autoimmune Diseases

Approximately 3–5% of the world population has at least one of more than 60 autoimmune conditions, and the figure rises to 5–8% in countries like the United States. According to the World Health Organization, the prevalence of these diseases appears to be increasing. Autoimmune diseases can arise at any time throughout life beginning with neonatal-onset diseases like Kawasaki disease up to diseases that frequently occur later in life such as rheumatoid arthritis (RA) and lupus. However, these usually adult-onset diseases are being seen more in children in the forms of juvenile idiopathic arthritis and pediatric-onset lupus. Even if these illnesses occur later in life, usually the groundwork for the immune system disruption was already laid during pregnancy, early life and childhood. In fact, autoimmune diseases generally occur in conditions where appropriate immune regulation breaks down.

There are at least two developmental routes to autoimmune disease. The first involves interference with the thymus during its prenatal role in establishing the immune repertoire among T cells. Instead of removing T cells that will cause autoimmunity, the damaged thymus allows them to persist after birth. A second route to autoimmunity involves interference with T regulatory cells (Tregs) whose job it is to prevent autoimmune responses. Other changes in specific organs, like the inappropriate activation of brain macrophages (such as microglia) due to environmental insult, may also be important in promoting specific autoimmune diseases. Certain infections, like hepatitis A or B virus infection that precedes autoimmune hepatitis, can compromise body tissues and may increase the likelihood of autoimmune responses in individuals with certain genetic backgrounds.

Some diseases listed under the autoimmune label are more complex. For example, celiac disease is not only an autoimmune disease but also has allergic disease elements as well. Its most prominent feature is an allergic reaction to a protein found in gluten (a substance found in wheat and other grain products). The initial allergic reaction progresses to autoimmune inflammation of the G.I. tract in which the body attacks its own gut tissue. So this disease spans both the category of an autoimmune disease and of an allergic disease.

One important feature of autoimmune diseases is that they tend to show a significant gender-bias. That is, a single disease is often more prevalent in one gender (e.g., females) than the other. Most autoimmune diseases show a female bias, however, some like alkylosing spondylitis show a male predominance. From the point of view of the immune system, the gender-bias is most likely a reflection of the nature of the environmental factor that was encountered (e.g., a chemical that can mimic estrogen), the genetic makeup of the child, the timing of the environmental exposure (e.g., third trimester pregnancy vs. after birth), and the levels of sex hormones in the child's system both at the time of exposure and in later life.

Autoimmune diseases that are reported to be promoted by early-life, environmental immune insult are: autoimmune thyroiditis (Hashimoto's and Grave's disease), autoimmune myocarditis, celiac disease (both adult and pediatric), Crohn's disease, inflammatory bowel disease (IBD),

Kawasaki disease, multiple sclerosis (MS), rheumatoid arthritis (RA, both adult and juvenile forms), scleroderma, Sjögren's disease, lupus and type 1 diabetes. Some of these diseases are promoted by the same type of immune dysfunction, and the diseases may be found to coexist in patients later in life (e.g., type 1 diabetes with later-life celiac and/or RA). Others, such as lupus, appear to result from different types of immune dysfunctions. For instance, RA is promoted by misdirected Th1 responses while lupus is promoted by misdirected Th2 responses. Because of this, it is rare for RA and lupus to coexist.

Unfortunately, the environmental risk factors for autoimmune diseases are less well defined than they are for allergic diseases. However, they do include certain environmental chemicals, drugs, diet and infections. Those factors that have been identified or suggested to promote an increased risk of autoimmunity are: mercury, diethylstilbestrol (DES), tobacco smoke, alcohol and recreational drugs, some medications used to induce immunosuppression such as cyclophosphamide and cyclosporin A, dioxin and certain infections.

Cardiovascular Diseases

Cardiovascular diseases connected to an early-life immune insult fall into two general categories. The first was already mentioned in the previous section and concerns autoimmune responses that affect the cardiovascular system. Autoimmune myocarditis in children belongs in this category. However, a second major category concerns misregulated inflammation (inflammation that occurs either when it shouldn't or more intensely and widespread in the body than is useful). This second category of inappropriate responses is caused by the major inflammatory cells — macrophages and neutrophils.

Overproduction of tissue-damaging oxygen radicals and excessive, misregulated production of nitric oxide (NO) are common occurrences after an early-life immune insult. In addition to weakening the heart and vasculature (veins and arteries), these types of dysfunctions are also connected to cardiac disease, particularly atherosclerosis. In fact, dysfunctional macrophages taking on the role of "foam cells" are literally sitting at the heart of arthlerosclerotic plaques in the arteries. Their misregulation and inappropriate responses to their environment and daily life are central to this disease. While a majority of atherosclerosis cases appear in adulthood, the immune dysfunction connected to the disease may be linked to a prenatal or neonatal environmental insult.

Some suggested risk factors for early-life immune insult involved in cardiovascular disease are: maternal diet during pregnancy and prenatal exposure to metals such as arsenic. Considering the fact that arsenic levels in drinking water have now been linked to later-life diabetes, arsenic may be of a greater concern than was once supposed.

Childhood Cancers

Cancers develop due to the uncontrolled replication of cells (because of mutagens, genetic susceptibility, etc.) and the inability of the immune system to rein in the growth of those cells. Impaired immunity against tumors due to immune system dysfunction can elevate the risk of cancer. This type of immune system dysfunction can affect the susceptibility of developing cancer over a lifetime. Amazingly, tumor immunity can be impacted by similar early-life immune insults to those affecting the risk of allergic and infectious diseases. For this reason, the status of the developing immune system during pregnancy and infancy is a major concern. Additionally, cancer can be caused by a dysfunctional immune system that produces chronic inflammation. The immune system becomes constantly activated as if it is always fighting a major infection, even if it's not. At this point, the immune system produces toxic by-products designed to kill bacteria. However, in the absence of any foreign bacteria, it can cause cells to mutate and become cancerous. For this reason it is not surprising that in diseases featuring a constantly activated immune system and chronic inflammation (e.g., ME/chronic fatigue syndrome), cancer is a leading cause of death.

During childhood, the predominant form of cancer that research has linked to immune system dysfunction is childhood acute lymphoblastic leukemia (cALL). In this disease, the data suggest that a dysfunctional immune response to a common childhood pathogen(s), such as a bacterial or viral infection, is a final step leading to leukemia. In order for the dysfunctional immune response to come into play in childhood, some early environmental modification of the developing immune system had to have occurred. Genetic background sets the stage in determining which children will be most susceptible. But an environmental insult usually works with the genetic predisposition to create the conditions for a child to develop the disease. While definite environmental factors have yet to be established, some are coming to the forefront as likely offenders, such as: maternal smoking during pregnancy and exposure to second hand smoke, maternal diet during pregnancy, and exposure to certain pesticides, radiation, jet fuel, strong electromagnetic fields.

Neurological Diseases

The neurological system seems to be particularly vulnerable to early life environmental insults. Brain macrophages, known as microglia and astrocytes, can cause local tissue damage if they are inappropriately activated or if their inflammatory responses aren't sufficiently controlled. Problems can occur during pregnancy if the mother has certain infections (such as influenza) or if chemicals she's exposed to damage or activate these cells in the fetus. There is also a concern that autoantibody production directed against targets in the brain may result.

Diseases that research has linked to early-life inflammation and/or immune insults include attention deficit disorder, autism spectrum disorders (ASDs), schizophrenia, Parkinson's disease and now Alzheimer's. In the cases of diseases of aging, an early-life immune assault to portions of the brain can cause cellular damage that, with normal aging, appear as neurological deficits and disease later in life. Take the example of Parkinson's disease. A prenatal immune assault on the brain often reduces the number of dopamine receptors available. Later in life, when dopamine receptors are being pared back as a natural process of aging, the brain suddenly has too few dopamine receptors and the symptoms of Parkinson's disease become apparent.

In children, diagnoses of autism and ASDs have exploded in sheer numbers and early-life environmental risk factors are thought to be involved. Children with these conditions frequently show signs of immune dysfunction that may also include gastrointestinal inflammation. The question is whether a prenatally-induced immune dysfunction might be a causative factor in the neurological condition, or whether the resulting immune dysfunction is simply an associated outcome that occurs as part of the overall toxicological response. More research will need to be performed before the determination between these possibilities can be made.

The identified and suspected risk factors for neurological conditions to date are: heavy metal exposures (lead, mercury), certain pesticides, volatile organic chemicals and certain maternal infections during pregnancy.

Infectious Diseases and Adverse Vaccine Responses

As any parent knows, infectious diseases are a normal part of childhood. But prenatal and neonatal immune insults can create problems with the child's ability to respond to and resist infections. In turn, this reduced ability to fight off infections can jeopardize a child's survival or lead to a parade of infections that require an excessive use of antibiotics early in life. The risk of acquiring an infection begins at birth with possible challenges such as neonatal sepsis. The risks continue as the infant and toddler face respiratory viruses, gastrointestinal pathogens, pathogens with neural targets (e.g., meningitis) and opportunistic infections (viral — disseminated cytomegalovirus, bacterial — some mycobacteria infections [the same category of bacteria as causes TB], protozoan parasites — cryptosporidium, fungal — Candida infections). Most children will be exposed to these infectious agents. The issue is whether their immune systems will be prepared to fight off the spectrum of potential infections.

The whole problem with infectious diseases is due to fact that the newborn's innate immune system is relatively immature. It needs exposure to pieces of bacteria in order to develop and mature fully. Additionally, the antiviral arm of the immune response, which is driven by mature dendritic cells along with Th1 cells, must increase in capacity immediately after birth. These changes must occur rapidly for the child's immune system to be able to effectively resist the mix of pathogens present in the environment. Certain immune insults prior to birth can block this maturation process and shift the immune system into a state that increases the child's risk for chronic and/or life-threatening diseases. Beyond neonatal sepsis, susceptibility to ear infections, including otitis media, is likely if innate immunity and Th1 activity fail to mature adequately.

And it isn't a coincidence that susceptibility to otitis media and allergic disease go hand-in-hand. Both are likely where innate immunity and Th1 levels are under-developed leaving a fetal freeze state where Th2 driven responses and misregulated inflammation predominate.

A further problem with early-life immune insult and risk of infectious disease concerns the effectiveness of childhood vaccinations. They are a boon to society's health in helping to eradicate some of the deadliest diseases of childhood and beyond. However, as more is becoming known about the development of the immune system, both prenatally and in the first few years of life, it is becoming increasingly obvious that there is a delicate balancing act that must be established when giving vaccinations in order to provide the greatest protection while not creating further problems.

For one, it's imperative that the child's immune system be sufficiently matured after birth in order to respond adequately to a vaccine. If the vaccinations are given too soon, and the child's immune system is not sufficiently developed, the vaccination could actually create health problems rather than conferring immunity.

For another, it's important to know whether the child's immune system was impaired in some way during the pregnancy. In cases where children were exposed during pregnancy to an immunotoxicant such as PCBs, childhood vaccine response can be so poor that children are not protected against those diseases even after boosters. This was seen in the Faroe Islands where the largely marine diet led to high PCB exposures for both the developing fetus and nursing children. A collaborative study of Faroe Island mothers and their children conducted by researchers at the University of South Denmark and the Harvard University School of Public Health found that PCB exposure levels at birth predicted the vaccine responses of the children when they were age seven. The researchers tested cord blood levels of PCBs then followed the children through their vaccination regimens. What they found was that the higher the cord blood levels of PCBs had been, the less likely vaccinations were to have conferred immunity. In other words, even though the children had received their shots and boosters, many weren't adequately protected against the diseases for which they had been vaccinated. This example shows why it's important to manage the prenatal and neonatal environment for the child to have optimal health later on.

Table 10.1. Environmental risk factors during pregnancy that are thought to increase the risk of childhood infectious diseases.

Maternal smoking	Tributyltin compounds (e.g., protective wood preservative)
Maternal alcohol intake	Endocrine disruptors (e.g., bisphenol A)
Recreational drugs	Certain pesticides (e.g., chlordane, heptachlor, methoxychlor)
PCBs	Polycyclic aromatic hydrocarbons (in BBQ smoke, surface run off from roads, industrial sewage, fossil fuel combustion)
Dioxin	Specific maternal dietary fat intake
Heavy metals (e.g., lead, mercury, cadmium)	Trichloroethylene (e.g., dry cleaning and industrial fluids)

As previously mentioned for dioxin, model studies suggest that prenatal exposure to the chemical causes both immunosuppression and misregulated inflammation. So simultaneously one part of the immune system is being suppressed while another part is being revved up and producing toxic metabolites (e.g., hydrogen peroxide). This seemingly impossible combination of suppression and activation is seen in individuals whose immune systems were damaged early on. A case of misregulated inflammation can actually cause a viral infection, such as influenza, to be more damaging to airways since the misguided response tends to damage the local tissue rather than clear the virus.

Some protection or enhanced resistance to infections has been reported when a newborn is exposed to an environment that includes animals and bacteria components. This is part of what has become known as the "hygiene hypothesis," which is covered in Chapter 21. The immune enhancement concerns the potential benefit of a newborn to being exposed to a non-sterile environment. Research studies seem to show that early postnatal exposure to some bacteria helps the immature immune system to mature more completely, better enabling it to meet the onslaught of childhood infections. This has led to the general concept that a completely sterile environment (one that is scrubbed thoroughly, often with antibacterial soaps) is actually not best for a newborn. In order for the newborn's immune system to learn, grow and mature, it needs a world filled with a bit of (lead free) soil and microbes. An interesting note is the fact that the risk of allergic disease is also reduced when the newborn's immune system matures more completely. So by allowing the very young to be exposed to a less than sterile environment, it may be possible to protect them against allergies and to help their immune system mature enough to respond more robustly to the usual childhood infections.

Conclusions

You may have noticed by now that many of the same risk factors can be applied to different categories of diseases. One reason is that only a subset of chemicals and drugs have undergone extensive immunotoxicological screening, been evaluated for disease implications in animals studies and been analyzed in longitudinal human epidemiological studies. The reality is that there are likely to be many more factors yet to be identified. However, where toxins and dietary factors are capable of affecting multiple categories of disease through early-life exposure and immune dysfunction, the dysfunction in turn impacts multiple sectors of the immune system. An immune-based tendency toward allergic disease may also mean that an individual has an increased susceptibility for otitis media, later life lupus and certain infections because the same immune dysfunction is responsible. Simultaneously, that same individual probably has a lower risk for type 1 diabetes and vice versa.

Prenatal and neonatal immune insults are likely to promote multiple diseases. This further emphasizes the benefit of choosing prevention as a front-line strategy to address the chronic illnesses and conditions that are presently on the rise.

Overview of Diseases

- Immune dysfunction-based diseases are more diverse in nature and affect more children than previously recognized.
- Most of the diseases are chronic and require decades of constant medical treatment.
- Immune dysfunction-based diseases impair the quality of life of both children and adults.

Chapter 11 — The Disease Progression Matrix

Introduction

In the prior chapter we discussed the diseases associated with early-life exposure to toxins and other environmental conditions (e.g., stress) that result in immune dysfunction. Many of these diseases are serious. Most of them are chronic and require a lifetime of medical and pharmacological treatment. Virtually all of the diseases significantly affect quality of life.

The current chapter shows that these diseases do not occur in a vacuum. Instead, they are connected to each other via problems created by immune dysfunction. In fact, a significant percentage of the diseases and conditions our children will encounter both during childhood and as adults form part of an immune dysfunction web or matrix. This chapter illustrates the matrix and how we can use that information to better protect our children.

Groups of immune-related diseases share similar underlying causes. Most of the research to date has only examined two or three of these diseases at a time. For example, studies in epidemiology have asked whether children with hayfever or eczema are more likely to be diagnosed with asthma at a later time than children without hayfever or eczema. The answer is yes. But recently, use of very large medical databases has allowed better identification of more complex patterns of interconnected diseases. Those comparisons have provided some striking findings. 1) Diseases within a category (e.g., allergic diseases) tend to go together in children. This means that a child may get more than one disease in this category (allergic rhinitis and asthma). 2) Some categories of diseases (e.g., inflammatory or autoimmune) have unexpected secondary conditions associated with them. These may include: sleep problems, clinical depression, hearing loss and cancer.

Why is it important to identify a matrix of diseases? The answer is that diseases like childhood asthma, type 1 diabetes, celiac disease or inflammatory bowel disease are only the first ones in a likely progression of diseases over a child's lifetime. When a child is diagnosed with a specific immune-related pediatric disease or condition, we now know that the child has an increased risk of specific additional immune-related diseases. The hayfever-asthma connection was mentioned as one of these examples. That same allergic child also has either no additional risk or even a reduced risk of some other conditions. For example, childhood asthma and type 1 diabetes are diseases that tend to exclude each other rather than clustering together.

By identifying these immune disease patterns, we can provide even greater incentive and impetus for relevant safety testing that can help prevent the first childhood immunological disease in the sequence. Additionally, we can provide better clues to pediatricians for treatments that may address the initial disease in such a way as to lessen the risk of the later-life diseases.

Categories of Connected Diseases

In a recent review article, R. Dietert and J. Zelikoff (*Current Pediatric Reviews*) described a complex checkerboard of immune dysfunction-associated diseases. Some of them seem to develop from each other while others rarely tend to occur in the same child. The lineage of diseases in a matrix does not mean that a given child will necessarily develop more than one of the interconnected diseases. It simply means that once the first immune-related disease is diagnosed, the child has an increased risk for developing one or more of the related diseases at some point in life.

Here, rather than presenting this complex checkerboard, we will discuss the connected diseases as they are organized by four disease categories: allergic, autoimmune, inflammatory and infectious diseases.

These are not meant to cover every possible disease linkage. Instead, this illustrates the importance for parents and pediatricians to recognize that diagnosis of one immune-related disease or condition may mean that the child needs special attention in order to prevent the others. This is because the immune relationships data say this first childhood disease is likely to be an entryway to a string of later specific heath issues. Here are four disease matrix examples:

1. *Example of an Allergic Category Disease Matrix*

Primary Childhood Disease: Asthma

Secondary Diseases or Conditions: (Increased risk in children with asthma)

Atopic dermatitis (eczema)
Allergic rhinitis (hayfever)
Increased risk of respiratory infections including influenza
Otitis media (ear infections)
Olfactory dysfunction (inability to identify smells)
Obesity
Behavioral disorders
Urinary incontinence (women)
Lung cancer

2. *Example of an Autoimmune Category Disease Matrix*

Primary Childhood Disease: Type 1 Diabetes

Secondary Diseases or Conditions: (Increased risk in children with type 1 diabetes)

Autoimmune thyroiditis (Hashimoto's and Grave's Disease)
Celiac disease
Multiple sclerosis
Atherosclerosis
Depression
Hearing loss
Sleep problems (insomnia)

3. *Example of an Inflammatory Category Disease Matrix*

Primary Childhood Disease: Inflammatory Bowel Disease (IBD)

Secondary Diseases or Conditions: (Increased risk in children with IBD)

Rheumatoid arthritis
Multiple sclerosis
Autoimmune hepatitis
Ankylosing spondylitis (inflammatory arthritis which can lead to fusion of the spine)
Asthma
Polyneuropathy (many peripheral nerves throughout the body malfunction at the same time)
Pediatric deep vein thrombosis
Depression
Colorectal cancer

4. *Example of an Infectious Category Disease Matrix*

Primary Childhood Disease(s): Infant Respiratory Infection/Rhinitis

Secondary Disease or Conditions: (Increased risk in children with severe early-life infections/rhinitis)

Asthma
Otitis media (ear infections)
Chronic bronchitis
Secondary bacterial infections (e.g., bacterial pneumonia)
Atherosclerosis
Cerebral arteriopathy (a disease of brain blood vessels that can lead to childhood stroke)
Adult snoring
Lung cancer

What the Matrix of Diseases Teaches Us: Five Lessons

There are several take-home lessons we can learn from these disease associations.

Lesson 1: Allergic diseases cluster together

By looking at the asthma disease pattern, it is clear that other allergic conditions are quite likely to occur as secondary diseases. If we were to use hayfever as the primary disease, we would see similar results. Again, this is not a coincidence but, instead, reflects a common immune dysfunction where Th2 responses predominate and IgE is inappropriately produced.

Lesson 2: One autoimmune disease can often beget another

When type 1 diabetes and IBD occur in children, there is an increased risk of the child developing other autoimmune diseases. This is not a coincidence. The combination of environment and genetics that produces the first childhood autoimmune disease is also ready to produce other similar immune dysfunction-based diseases once the right trigger occurs (see the later chapter on causes and triggers). Essentially, it is only a matter of which organ and system will be affected. Therefore, the underlying immune dysfunction needs to be addressed to avoid the risk of additional autoimmune diseases later in life.

Lesson 3: Some primary diseases may be direct triggers of secondary diseases via tissue-damaging immune responses

This infectious disease category that begins with severe respiratory infections and rhinitis appears to be primarily focused on secondary diseases also occurring in the upper body. Many of these appear to be a result of inflammatory damage and injured tissue. This raises the question of whether the respiratory infectious agents are actually a cause of all these diseases or if, instead, they are a trigger that allows a dysfunctional immune system to cause damage and to produce additional diseases. This is discussed in detail in Chapter 18.

Lesson 4: Some childhood immune-related diseases cause specific tissue damage that can lead to later-life cancer in those tissues

Other possible surprises from the secondary disease lists are the reported higher risk of lung cancer among non-smoking asthmatics compared with other non-smokers, and the elevated risk of colorectal cancer among those with IBD. These later life diseases are actually logical if you realize that decades of asthma-associated inflammation in the lung and IBD in the G.I. tract can lead to a considerable amount of oxidative damage to cells in those tissues. Given enough time and persistent inflammation, cancer is a likely outcome.

Lesson 5: Misregulated inflammation, if not corrected, can produce serious depression

At first glance you may ask why clinical depression would occur in children with type 1 diabetes or inflammatory bowel disease? The fact is that inappropriate inflammation is a hallmark for both of these diseases along with additional autoimmune components. Other cases where misregulation of inflammation occurs also have clinical depression as a likely co-existing condition. For example, this occurs with multiple sclerosis and ME/CFS. Depression appears to go hand-in-hand with out of control inflammation-promoting cytokine production (e.g., IL-6). Note that sleep problems are also connected to inflammation problems, since the same cytokines can influence the neurological and endocrine systems.

Conclusions

The idea of discussing a matrix or a pattern of immune-related diseases is relatively new, but it is an idea that can be quite useful. The existence of patterns of immune-related diseases is increasingly supported by scientific studies, and the identification of specific patterns can be helpful in protecting the health of our children over a lifetime. When chemicals, drugs, diet, physical and psychological factors cause immune dysfunction, the perils are not restricted only to the earliest disease seen in childhood. Instead, there is a progression of specific diseases that is based on the type of immune dysfunction that is producing them. This means we have an even stronger obligation to identify early life immune hazards and to keep our children safe from them. Additionally, we need to ask physicians to consider treatment strategies for the long term. The best strategies should not only address the symptoms currently at hand. They should also consider the other diseases that may be sitting just over the horizon. Those diseases are already programmed to appear when triggered and can represent an additional health risk in the absence of effective childhood immune management.

Overview of Disease Matrices

- Immune dysfunction-related diseases occur in distinct clusters.
- Many childhood diseases (e.g., asthma, type 1 diabetes) are only the first in a predictable sequence of potential life-long diseases tied to the same underlying immune problem.
- Many diseases and conditions are not often recognized as being linked to childhood immune dysfunction (e.g., sleep disorders, metabolic problems, loss of senses-hearing, smell).

Chapter 12 — Categories of Environmental, Physical and Psychological Factors

Introduction

One of the goals of this book is to provide science-based information that can be useful in both practical day-to-day activities and for longer-term planning. Part of that information involves a discussion of some risk factors to avoid and some proactive factors to embrace. The proactive factors, which are presented in a later chapter, are all those activities (such as maternal and childhood diet) that have been shown to protect the child's immune system for functional balance and reduced risk of disease. These are steps that can be taken representing one side of the coin in optimizing your child's chances for immune health.

However, there is another side of the child's immune system coin. That involves all the potential hazards for the developing immune system. These hazards include environmental exposures, therapeutics, physical factors, psychological factors and biological conditions that contribute to immune problems in childhood. Many of these are well established for harming the immune system at exposures that you or your child are likely to encounter in real life. For other hazards, newer research suggests we need to pay closer attention to them.

It is important that we first discuss the categories of factors that can affect the immune system both positively and negatively. These are the names and technical terms that parents may see appearing in magazines, newspapers and on the Internet. Some may be familiar like heavy metals and diet while others with names like "endocrine disruptors" or "volatile organic compounds" may be less familiar. These are presented to: 1) help parents understand what chemicals, drugs, dietary factors, and physical and psychological stressors may fall within these commonly used categories and 2) illustrate the breadth of the factors that can affect your child's immune system.

In Chapter 16, the "Top 25 Risk Factors" for your child's immune system are discussed. These are the high priority hazards to be aware of and avoid if possible. Chapter 17 and the Appendix present additional immune risk factors beyond the Top 25. Chapter 20 discusses some positive factors (e.g., dietary antioxidants) for consideration during the prenatal and childhood periods of immune development. Of course, whether a factor is helpful or a problem for the child's immune system can be influenced by the dose of the exposure or the amount ingested through diet. This was discussed in the previous "Toxicology 101" chapter and will be considered again in both the Diet and the Hygiene chapters.

Categories of Risk Factors for the Prenatal and Childhood Immune System

Alcohol

Alcohol is thought to play a significant role both as a prenatal immunotoxicant (via maternal exposure) and as a problem in later childhood. The risks associated with prenatal exposure are discussed in the Top 25 Risks chapter. Alcohol consumption by adolescents and teens is considered to be a postnatal risk factor for autoimmune disease. We discuss this more in the chapter on postnatal triggers of diseases.

Childhood Infections and Vaccinations

Childhood infections play an important role in immune-related diseases. In particular, they are of interest as potential factors in both autoimmune diseases as well as some forms of childhood leukemia. Additionally, possible health risks associated with vaccinations have emerged as a concern among many parents. These topics are considered in the chapter on postnatal triggers of disease.

Dietary Factors

Diet is an important consideration for the immune system both during prenatal development and nursing and during later childhood. Among dietary factors is the issue of prenatal undernutrition, which can dramatically affect birth parameters and the risk of later life disease. Beyond that is the potential for food contamination by toxic chemicals. Many of these toxins such as pesticides, mold toxins, and industrial chemicals are discussed in later chapters.

The composition of the diet is important as well. Amino acid balance can affect immune cells, their maturation and their metabolism. Protein sources can also affect production of such critical factors as nitric oxide. Some dietary proteins (e.g., the proteins in nuts, cow's milk and shellfish) can serve as food allergens. These are important as well.

Dietary fatty acids (e.g., omega-3 fatty acids) are critical determinants in the control of inflammation. Both maternal and neonatal fatty acid intake can affect immune-based disease risk for years to come and are discussed in Chapter 20. Similarly, dietary estrogen-like chemicals can also influence immune status. Genistein, a component of soy, is included among later chapters.

Finally, micronutrients and vitamins are of major importance. Many are needed to sustain cells and to facilitate detoxification of harmful chemicals and drugs. As previously mentioned, some micronutrients such as selenium can themselves be toxins when the dietary or supplemental intake is too high. But selenium deficiency also places a child's immune system in jeopardy. These factors are considered in more depth in later chapters.

Drugs of Abuse

Most known drugs of abuse are potent toxins for the immune system, and children are more sensitive than adults. Among the drugs that have been most extensively studied for developmental immunotoxicity (DIT) are cocaine, marijuana, methamphetamine and the opioids. Two of these are discussed in the "Top 25 Risks" chapter.

Immune cells are sensitive to these chemicals because they have receptors on the cell surfaces for many of them. As occurs with other categories of chemicals, modulation of the immune cells during critical windows of development can cause problems that are much more extensive and longer lasting than similar exposures would be in adults.

Endocrine-Disrupting Chemicals

The general category consisting of endocrine-disrupting chemicals (EDCs) covers a wide variety of chemicals in the environment. It represents environmental contaminants, foodstuffs and drugs. The category is # 3 on the Top 25 List because EDCs include an extensive list of chemicals and drugs that would-be-parents and children are likely to encounter. Many EDCs are discussed within this section while some other toxicants that have EDC activity have their own section later in the Top 25 List (e.g., lead, mercury, dioxin, PCBs).

EDCs have the capacity to alter hormone balance and/or to bind to hormone receptors and produce a change. EDCs include environmental estrogens as well as those chemicals that are anti-androgens (chemicals that block testosterone production or use in the body). While much of the focus has been on synthetic chemicals in the environment, EDCs are also found in foods like baby formula. Pregnant women and new parents need to be aware of the sources of EDCs and their potential impact on the developing immune system.

One of the reasons why the immune system is so sensitive to EDCs is because many immune cells have receptors for a variety of hormones including estrogen. As a result, the development and function of immune cells can be directly impacted by the level and balance of hormones in the body. When the balance is shifted inappropriately during critical maturational steps of immune system development, the effects may be more profound and longer-lasting than might otherwise be expected. Additionally, the effects of exposure to EDCs are likely to be different in female vs. male babies. So, attention to the intake of and the exposure to EDCs can be a considerable benefit to your baby's immune system and overall health.

Halogenated Aromatic Hydrocarbons (HAHs)

The HAHs are both man-made and naturally occurring. They contain some of the most significant toxins for the immune and reproductive systems. Among these are the dioxins and polychlorinated biphenyls (PCBs), which are discussed in the Top 25 List. This category also includes the polybrominated biphenyls (PBBs).

These chemicals are produced in a wide variety of industrial activities and significant prior pollution has been deposited in our environment. Additionally, these are persistent pollutants in that they take a long time to decay. It takes about a decade for half the concentration of these pollutants to be broken down in the environment. They are also stored in the fat tissue of exposed humans and animals. These chemicals are among the most potent immunotoxicants known and are particularly important during early life exposure.

Heavy Metals

Heavy metals are the general name given to several metallic elements with higher molecular weights (at least five times that of water) in the chemical periodic table. They include lead, mercury, cadmium and arsenic. The developing immune system is quite sensitive to toxicity from heavy metals, and each metal produces a spectrum of adverse effects that appear to overlap with the adverse effects produced by other heavy metals.

Hygiene

The newborn's immune system is relatively immature at birth and must mature rapidly to meet the challenges that are ahead for the child. Recently, scientists have suggested that a completely aseptic environment missing some level of exposure to microbes along with animals is unhelpful for immune maturation. Some evidence supports the possible benefits of exposure to farm animals and/or pets and their inherently less than sterile environment in reducing the risk of childhood asthma and allergies. This topic is discussed in Chapter 21, the "Hygiene and Pets" chapter.

Maternal Infections

Infection during pregnancy can result in maternal immune activation. This can create cytokine imbalances and inflammation in the developing fetus. The impact of the immune activation seems to play out in a variety of organs. But much of the focus has been on immune-activation-mediated damage to the brain.

The level of concern for the developing baby depends upon the type of infection and the stage of the pregnancy. With some maternal infections during pregnancy, fetal brain inflammation may occur. This may elevate the risk of certain neurological conditions such as schizophrenia, epilepsy and possibly even autism. Maternal influenza infection during pregnancy has also been associated with Attention Deficit Hyperactivity Disorder (ADHD) in children for at least the last decade. Infections during pregnancy are not always possible to avoid. But parents-to-be may want to do what they can in working with their OB/GYN to minimize the risk.

Mold (Fungal) Toxins

Several types of fungi produce metabolites that are potent toxins for the immune system as well as other physiological systems (e.g., respiratory, neurological, gastrointestinal). These are also known as mycotoxins. One category of these chemicals called the Trichothecenes contains four subtypes (A–D) that differ in exact chemical structure. These toxins are naturally-occurring where molds grow, and some have been adapted for specialized medical use while others have been used in chemical warfare. Those mold toxins of greatest concern in food are among Types A and B while Type D contains the famous black mold toxins that often contaminate the interior of houses and office buildings. These are covered in more detail in a later chapter.

Nutraceuticals

Nutraceuticals are foods or dietary supplements that are given to promote health and/or prevent specific diseases. This category includes a variety of herbal- and fungal-derived medicines that have significant potential to affect the immune system. As with other dietary factor or drugs, the dose is important in both the safety and effectiveness of nutraceuticals. Examples of these would be Panax ginseng, green tea and Echinacea extract. These are discussed in both Chapter 15 and in Chapter 20.

Pesticides and Herbicides

Pesticides and herbicides have been under scrutiny for years for the possibility of contributing to human health problems. However, with the organochlorine and organophosphate pesticides, more of the focus has been on risk of neurotoxicity rather than immunotoxicity. Among these pesticides, those known to produce significant DIT problems are: chlordane, heptachlor, and methoxyclor. These differ significantly in outcome depending upon the sex of the offspring. Why? Well, a variety of pesticides and herbicides have endocrine disrupting activity, and some of them may exert negative actions by interacting with endocrine receptors on immune cells. One category of anti-mollusk chemicals, the organotins, has shown potent developmental immunotoxicity. Exposure to organotins has been reported to cause the thymus to shrink during critical periods of immune development. Organotins were used historically in marine paints and as a wood preservative. Among the herbicides, the one of greatest interest is the heavily used atrazine. This chemical is discussed in detail in the "Top 25 Risk Factors."

Polycyclic Aromatic Hydrocarbons (PAHs)

The PAHs occur naturally in oil, coal and tar deposits. They are also the products of incomplete combustion whether from burning fossil fuel or organic materials (e.g., firewood). They also occur with roofing tar, asphalt, creosote, automobile exhaust, charbroiled meat and cigarette smoke. Examples of PAHs are the chemicals benzo[a]pyrene, dimethylbenzanthracene and 3-methylcholanthene. All three of these PAHs are potent immunotoxicants affecting both the developing and adult immune systems.

Stress and Trauma

Stress is among the most important factors in immune dysfunction. Sometimes it is difficult to fully appreciate the extent to which stress and/or trauma can impact immune function and inflammation. There are several reasons for this. First, stress can come from a variety of sources. There is physical stress as may occur with athletes in training or the stress from chronic abuse. Psychological stress can arise anytime in life and has multiple initiators. This category of stress can be worse than physical stress. Second, chemical/dietary stress affects multiple physiological systems including the immune system. Finally, microbial-associated stress can trigger unexpected immune-related diseases through inappropriate activation of the immune system or misdirected responses. These different causes of stress can follow overlapping biochemical pathways that extend through the immune, neurological and endocrine systems as well as the liver. Stress is considered in the following "Top 25 Risks" chapter but is also mentioned in the chapter on postnatal triggers of disease.

Tobacco Smoke

Tobacco smoke coming largely from cigarettes represents one of the most significant and preventable risk factors for the developing immune system. It is at the top of the list in the "Top 25 Risks" chapter that follows.

Therapeutic Drugs

Women who suffer from autoimmune diseases or cancer or who have received an organ transplant may have been administered immunosuppressive drugs as part of their therapy. This could include drugs such as cyclophosphamide, prednisone, dexamethasone, busulfan, cyclosporine A, FK-506, azathioprine and tacrolimus. Some of these drugs can cross the placenta or be transferred during nursing and can cause problems for the baby's immune system. Parents will want to check with their OB/GYN, pediatrician and pharmacist concerning the latest information regarding the specific drugs administered and the likelihood of transfer to the baby. Most studies have only asked whether the women had full term pregnancies. Questions of whether the offspring of women taking these drugs have a higher risk for allergic or autoimmune diseases were probably not investigated during the research, development and manufacture of these drugs.

Other therapeutic drugs designed for other purposes may or may not have been tested directly for risk of immune-based diseases in children. Parents should never hesitate to ask their physicians or pharmacists if this information exists in the safety records.

Volatile Organic Compounds (VOCs)

VOCs are a category that includes any organic chemical that under normal conditions can easily vaporize into air. This means that outside of occupational exposures to the chemicals as liquids or through hazardous spills, most people will encounter VOCs in the air in confined spaces (home, car, office). VOCs are an important component of indoor air pollution. Their maximum concentration is often much greater indoors than outside. Occasionally, they are found as drinking water contaminants usually as a result of prior industrial use in the area.

VOCs are thought to be a factor in sick building syndrome. They are emitted from a variety of sources including building materials, wood and laminated furniture, new carpets, photocopiers, shelving, plastics, cosmetics and paint strippers. Some specialized work areas such as beauty salons can have significant VOC emissions from the products that are used. Among the VOCs of greatest interest for children's health are formaldehyde, styrene, toluene, benzene and xylene.

Conclusions

Information in this chapter has set the stage for consideration of the most significant toxins for the developing immune system as well as those factors that are useful for protecting childhood immunity. These categories have basically defined our playing field for the child's immune system. Now the job is to find a useful balance of avoidance, prevention and proactive planning for the child's immune system. The chapters in Part III provide the necessary details about these factors that were used to develop an integrated strategy of immune protection.

Overview of Categories of Factors

- More categories exists of factors impacting the developing immune system than are usually discussed in individual publications (e.g., newspaper articles, science articles).
- They include:
  - — Environmental chemicals
  - — Drugs
  - — Physical factors (e.g., UV radiation, pathogens)
  - — Psychological factors (stress, trauma)
  - — Diet and supplements
  - — Hygiene
  - — Pets

Part II — Specific Strategies

Chapter 13 — Prenatal Strategies for Preventing Immune System Damage

Introduction

Part I of the book presented the basic science behind the developing immune system, the environmental factors that affect it and health risks that can result from early-life immune insult. Part III of the book and the Appendix will expand on the previous category of factors and their effects on the child's immune system. This section (Part II), with its three chapters, is the core of the book. In fact, it could be the reason you are awake and still reading. It provides the specific strategies that can be used to minimize the risk of immune damage and to increase the likelihood your child will develop a well-functioning immune system.

The present chapter considers preparation for the prenatal period while the following chapter covers the child's infant and adolescent stages of life. The material is presented as potential actions for parents and parents-to-be to use while working with their physician.

Not every set of parents will face the same exact set of environmental challenges for their baby's immune system. Nor is every environmental factor of equal significance for the developing immune system. But having in hand a practical guide or checklist of possible sources of both harmful and helpful environmental factors (e.g., toxic chemicals, drugs, dietary factors) and the situations in which they might be encountered is key to putting a strategy into place for managing your baby's immune system. Some potential sources of immune-altering environmental factors that are important during prenatal immune development are listed in this chapter. These sources and factors are of significance for your baby's developing immune system and are either well-established or highly suspected to affect immune development.

Personal Behavior and Choices

Avoid Maternal Smoking and Environmental Tobacco Smoke (ETS)

Tobacco smoke affects several different critical windows during prenatal and postnatal immune development. Both exposure from smoke directly inhaled by the pregnant woman and second-hand smoke from others are serious risks for the baby's immune, respiratory and cardiovascular systems. Avoidance of tobacco smoke is both possible and necessary. If the mother and/or father smoke, quitting with the help of your doctor before attempting to have a child is of paramount importance. However, once a pregnancy is discovered, quitting smoking is an absolute necessity to prevent immune damage and problems with other physical systems. Also, the pregnant mother should avoid places where others are smoking or ask that they refrain in her presence. While this could make for some less comfortable social situations, the benefits in protecting the unborn child's health far outweigh the discomfort.

Minimize/Avoid Maternal Alcohol Consumption

Exposing the fetus to alcohol is a serious concern for the immune system. It can cause increased susceptibility to infectious diseases and reduced innate immunity. While there may be a very low level of alcohol consumption that is safe, we don't know the "safe" level for each period of prenatal immune development. Other physiological systems are also affected by maternal alcohol intake. Therefore, minimizing, if not abstaining, from alcohol is the most protective route for fetal immune development. Some chemicals in grapes (e.g., resveratrol) have antioxidant activities and can be useful. But these can be obtained via grapes, grape juice and grape extracts without exposing your baby to the harmful effects of alcohol.

Minimize Stress During the Pregnancy

Stress that is intense and/or prolonged during pregnancy can negatively affect the developing immune system of the baby as well as other physiological systems. Often, reducing stress is easier said than done. However, a first step is to be aware that significant stress has the ability to make an imprint on the baby's immune system and to change your child's immune function for life. Increased stress can arise through many different sources linked to changes in family and home, the workplace, finances or even hormone balance. Certain techniques exist that may be helpful to manage stress such as meditation, yoga, Emotional Freedom Technique (EFT) and biofeedback. It may be useful to discuss stress and ways to manage it better with your physician and/or alternative complementary medicine practitioner.

If the expectant mother finds herself experiencing intense, acute stress (e.g., death of a loved one, partner's severe illness), reaching out to a qualified mental health care provider to support and help her through that difficult time does more than just improve her mental health and make the trauma easier to bear. Getting adequate mental health care while undergoing a trauma can mean the difference in how severely the stress impacts the developing baby.

Avoid the Use of Recreational Drugs

Obviously, the use of recreational drugs poses a serious concern for the prenatal immune system as well as for the neurological system. Immune cells have receptors for most drugs of abuse and can be affected by direct exposure to them. The drugs can severely impair the developing immune system and should be avoided. If the pregnant mother has used recreational drugs for a long time, she should seek medical help to quit as soon as possible.

Minimize Maternal Infections

Maternal infections are not really avoidable. However, the risk of certain infections can be affected by exposure to other infected individuals. Parents-to-be should be aware that if they minimize the incidence of certain infections during the pregnancy, the risk of inflammatory damage to the baby's immune and neurological systems will be greatly decreased. This may mean being less social during pregnancy, avoiding large crowds and small children. Take more precautions to reduce spread, such as washing your hands often and wiping down the handles on grocery store carts and in public restrooms.

Examine the Method of Birth Delivery Options

The method of birth delivery is often a medical decision that should be made by physicians. However, parents should be aware that vaginal delivery appears to offer advantages over Caesarian section for the baby's immune system. Vaginal delivery seems to promote an improved immune balance in the baby and may help jumpstart the immune system's maturation process. Therefore, if a Caesarian delivery is not a medical necessity, and the parents have options based on the physician's recommendations, vaginal delivery may be the better option for the baby's immune system.

Review Maternal Medications for Prenatal Immune Safety

Any medications taken during the pregnancy whether prescribed or over-the-counter should be discussed with your physician. However, parents-to-be should be aware that a number of prescription and over-the-counter medications can affect the developing immune system. This includes steroids (e.g., prednisone), antibiotics and non-steroidal anti-inflammatory drugs (NSAIDs such as Motrin, Advil and Aleve).

Parents need to ask their physician what safety data exist concerning the protection of the baby's immune system. If safety data do not yet exist for the pregnancy phase of a child's life, it may be best for the baby's immune system to refrain from taking the medication. Obviously, if the mother has an acute illness and needs the medication, then she and the doctor should work out the dose and length of time on the medication in order to minimize its impact on the developing child.

However, if it's a headache you're dealing with, you may consider trying some gentle stretching exercise, rest, or another alternative measure in order to deal with the pain (barring a migraine). If it's muscle aches, pregnancy massage can be an amazing blessing. The most important thing to do is to weigh the discomfort against the possible damage a medication can do before taking it and discuss the options with your physician.

Examine Dietary Intake and Use of Supplements

Maternal diet can be an important source of both helpful and harmful chemicals for the developing immune system. Intake of omega-3 fatty acids, zinc, vitamin D, and antioxidants such as selenium, vitamin E, vitamin C and pantothentic acid are important for immune development. Amino acid balance affected by different protein sources can also affect the prenatal immune system. Oral exposure to heavy metals such as mercury, lead and arsenic as well as polychlorinated biphenyls (PCBs) is a significant immunological concern. Both mercury and PCBs can be found in some larger species of fish, such as tuna and salmon. On-the-one-hand, the omega-3 fatty acids derived from fish are a necessity; on-the-other-hand, mercury and PCBs need to be avoided. Pregnant women need to scrutinize ways to get the fatty acids that they and their baby need while avoiding the toxic contaminants.

Home Environment and Neighborhood

Check the History of Properties in the Area for Past Industrial Use

The property where you live or intend to live along with its surrounding neighborhood has a history. And the result of certain histories has the ability to affect your baby's developing immune system. Many past industrial sites with heavy toxic contamination of soil and water have been identified and are likely to be known by residential communities. But smaller sites with spills, prior industrial waste disposal or inadvertent chemical contamination may either not be known or may not be well publicized. It is worth investigating what was done since the industrial revolution in the area where you will bring up your baby. This category of concern extends for both the prenatal and postnatal periods of development.

Among the immunotoxicants found at some sites are heavy metals, PCBs and trichloroethylene. Many sites have a mixture of several toxic chemicals. Because toxic chemical contamination can affect entire neighborhoods, knowing about your house, apartment, condominium or rental property alone may not tell you everything about the risk of exposure during pregnancy. It is worth knowing what is in the water and soil in the town where you and your baby will live.

Avoid/Minimize Hazardous Exposure With Home Renovations

Home renovation is often a part of welcoming a new baby into your life. When changes to houses or buildings are involved, this invariably leads to chemical and allergen exposures that are beyond those of everyday life. With older houses or buildings, increased exposure to some hazardous chemicals and/or allergens is virtually guaranteed. While the levels may not present an immediate hazard for your immune system, the same may not be true for your baby's developing immune system. If you are pregnant or anticipate that you may be in the near future, realize that home renovation may cause a significant release of heavy metals, volatile organic compounds, mycotoxins and allergens. Your exposure should be minimized whenever possible.

Additionally, toxins may be released as particles in the air and settle on surfaces to be present after the project is completed. Even changes to the exterior of houses can result in some soil contamination around the building. Home renovation-associated exposure to toxins and allergens may be one of the more common and under-appreciated risks for the developing immune system.

If home renovation before the baby comes is necessary, the expectant mother should not be involved in the actual work, particularly if the home was built before the mid-1970's when lead paints were frequently used. In fact, if any woodwork needs to be scraped and refinished, the mother would be safer to leave the house while the work was being done, have the house thoroughly cleaned for any dust residue and return only after both work and clean up are complete. We recognize such recommendations may not be easy to follow for many families. But they will help to reduce immunotoxic exposures when it is possible to implement them.

Check Household Products

One of the frequently overlooked sources of hazardous chemicals is the range of cleaning products, disinfectants, home maintenance products and personal care products around the house. Depending upon the exact products, they may contain toxic chemicals that can build up in the pregnant mother's body and pose a hazard for the baby's developing immune system.

For example, certain hair dyes, in particular brunette colors, include lead as do up to 75% of dark red lipsticks. Certain plastics used for food containers and food storage contain endocrine-disrupting toxins. Other products may contain pesticides, preservatives like formaldehyde or volatile organic compounds (VOCs). Safety levels of many of these chemicals may or may not have been directly established for the developing immune system.

It is useful to examine the chemicals in your arsenal of personal care, cleaning and disinfection products around the house to ensure that you maximize the safety of your baby's immune system during the pregnancy. Many "greener" products have recently come onto the market. These should offer a broader range of products available for comparison shopping. However, "greener" does not guarantee that a product is safer for the baby's immune system.

Check Chemicals Use in Neighborhood

Chemicals are often used to beautify or enhance the quality of properties including parks and public areas, as well as your neighbors' yards. These chemicals may be relatively safe for the developing immune system or not. Alternatively, they may never have been directly tested for impact on the developing immune system. Products may range from those intended for lawn care (e.g., weed killers) to those used for insect control. Some help to prevent diseases like those carried by mosquitoes. Using these chemicals may enhance the community's appeal and economic well-being. But as parents-to be, it is worth knowing what you and your baby's immune system may be exposed to through your own use of outdoor chemicals as well as that of your community.

Minimize Exposure to Traffic Pollution and Other Air Pollutants

Heavy traffic pollution is known to be an immunological concern both in prenatal and postnatal life. Exposure to other air pollutants such as wood smoke, air particles and gases can help produce oxygen radicals. Ozone pollution is also a risk for some cities and areas. This may be largely uncontrollable depending upon where a pregnant woman lives and works. However, it is useful to recognize this is one of the sources of immunotoxicants and that minimizing these exposures can benefit your baby's immune system.

One strategy with traffic pollution would be to keep the windows of the house on the roadway side closed. While this doesn't eliminate the threat, it can reduce your direct exposure to it.

Workplace Environment

Before and during the pregnancy a woman may spend a considerable amount of time in the workplace environment. The default assumption is usually that this workplace environment is completely safe, but that is not always the case. For example, even the Environmental Protection Agency once had a building in Washington, D.C. that was identified to produce "sick building syndrome." So no workplace facility is above scrutiny.

Many work facilities are closed environments so air quality including air exchange may help to determine the level of toxins present. Additionally, the location of air intake vents can be important as this is the source of fresh air for the building. If these vents are situated next to pollution sources such as parking lots or trash dumpsters, the air may not be as fresh as it appears. Toxins are not the only concern. If the air is cycled at a rate that is too slow, bacteria, viruses and allergens may also accumulate. Office equipment such as printers, copiers and even computers can contribute to the chemicals in the air and on surfaces. You may have carefully evaluated your household cleaning products for safety only to go to work and be exposed to the same toxic chemical products you just removed from your home.

Some additional jobs and workplaces may be associated with very specific occupational chemical exposures. While occupational exposure to hazardous chemicals is usually tightly regulated, safety levels may be set for the adult with little to no direct information available for impact on the developing immune system. So "safety first" should be a workplace motto that extends to your baby as well.

Conclusions

This chapter has presented certain strategies that parents can use to minimize harmful exposures and maximize the protective environment for the prenatal stages of a baby's immune development. Since this period appears to be the most sensitive to immune insult, the planning parents do before and during the pregnancy has the ability to affect the child's immune system throughout his or her lifetime. Not all of the steps are easy and some may be impractical depending upon individual circumstances. But knowing both the potential hazards and the immune-promoting factors can give parents better control of the interactions their baby's immune system has with the environment.

The next chapter will consider steps that are important for protecting the immune system of the newborn, infant and adolescent child. Not surprisingly, many of the same categories of harmful and helpful factors affect this period of a child's immune development as well. However, the relative importance among immune risk categories can change and some new ones appear on the horizon particularly for the newborn and toddler. So, onward to your new arrival.

Overview of Prenatal Strategies

- The prenatal period of immune development is the most sensitive for environmental disruption.
- Planning ahead to protect the developing immune system during the pregnancy may be the most effective step you can take to protect your child's immune system.

Chapter 14 — Strategies to Use During the First Few Years of Life

Introduction

If the prenatal period of development appears to be the most vulnerable for environmental insult of the developing immune system, then the next period of greatest concern for the child's immune system is the one immediately following birth and extending into adolescence. Most newborns are welcomed into the world possessing all of the immune cells needed for effective host defense but not all of the immune functional capacity they will need. Certain immune functions are blunted or skewed as part of the immune system's immaturity at birth. How quickly the immune system is able to complete its development and gain the balance of a mature system has a lot to do with the course of the child's health.

The child's parents have decisions to make and steps to take that can help to bring the baby's immune system into a more effective balance (one that is also dependent upon the genes the baby has inherited). In contrast, other decisions or options can have the effect of keeping the baby in a state of incomplete immune maturation similar to the state that was seen in utero. What the child is exposed to after birth can essentially "freeze" its immune system into a prolonged, immature imbalance and later immune dysfunction. Both innate immune responses and the balance of acquired responses are at risk. The child's immune system needs to mature quickly in order to face the disease challenges ahead.

Obviously, your child's immune system will continue to interact with the environment beyond the infant-to-toddler stages continuing through his/her teen years and beyond. Immune-promoting decisions will continue to serve your child's better health in those later years of childhood. But these early critical windows involve immune development, rather than the mere maintenance of an established immune system, and will set the template for your child's lifelong immune health.

General Considerations

Breastfeeding

One of the most beneficial activities for the newborn's immune system is breastfeeding. Of course breastfeeding provides the most natural nutrient source for babies, and it also allows the transfer of maternal antibodies that can afford protection against infections while the infant's immune system is undergoing steps in postnatal maturation. However, not everything about breastfeeding is beneficial. Many toxins the mother has ingested or inhaled are stored in fat. They can be released during breastfeeding and be transferred to the baby in the breast milk. These toxins and their transfer during nursing are of concern. However, in all but the most extreme circumstances of maternal toxicity, the benefits of breastfeeding for the baby's overall well-being and immune maturation appear to outweigh the concerns about contaminants in breast milk.

Soy-Based Formulas

Soy can provide isoflavones that can be helpful to the mature immune system. However, its use in formula appears to expose the newborn to endocrine-disrupting immunomodulators such as genistein. In other words, genistein makes undesirable changes to the developing immune system that increase the risk of immune dysfunction and immune-based diseases. Too much genistein is not a good thing for either the baby's immune system or its reproductive system. For this reason, care needs to be given when considering soy-based formulas as part of a baby's diet. If cow's milk allergy is the concern, a reasonable alternative might be a formula based on goat's milk.

Prebiotics

Prebiotics are complex carbohydrate substances found in nature (such as beta-glucans). They can promote the growth of probiotic bacteria in a baby's G.I. tract and appear to also help the baby's innate immune cells mature more effectively. It may be useful for parents to discuss the potential benefits of prebiotics with their pediatrician. Prebiotics may encourage the immune system within the baby's intestinal tract to mature efficiently as well.

Probiotics

Probiotics are generally friendly bacteria (such as those found in some yogurts) that take up residence in the G.I. tract of children and adults. They provide at least two benefits. They crowd out dangerous bacteria thereby reducing the chances of intestinal disease. They also alter metabolism in a way that may help to protect against certain food allergies. As with prebiotics, probiotics can help you manage your child's immune system and are worth examination.

Vaccinations

Vaccinations are an important part of preventing childhood disease and they work (see Chapter 19). Like many areas of life, some vaccines carry a small risk of side effects. But these are generally outweighed by the benefits of disease prevention. So vaccinations are, in general, a major and effective tool in the parent's arsenal against health risks for their child. Parents are urged to work with the pediatrician to protect their child against preventable childhood diseases. However, legitimate questions do exist about the optimum timing for childhood vaccinations in order to create the best outcome for the developing immune system. The timing of vaccines should be best for the child's overall health. This type of information needs to be available for all vaccines to reduce the potential risk of all immune-related diseases.

Parents need to be aware of recent research showing connections between the timing of vaccinations and other chronic conditions like asthma. Don't hesitate to bring articles and questions to your child's pediatrician and discuss what an optimum schedule of vaccination might look like for your child. You and your child's pediatrician should be partners in the care of your child's immune system.

Antibiotic and Medication Use

Use of medication and prescription antibiotics should be done under appropriate medical guidance. However, parents should be aware that overuse of antibiotics in children is a problem for the immune system. It is important to evaluate medical necessity with your pediatrician while the immune system is developing. Additionally, restoring the friendly gut bacteria in the G.I. tract following antibiotic use is necessary and, if the course of antibiotics has been for a long enough time, it can be critical. Other medications may present special health risks for the child. Be sure to ask your pediatrician if, and to what extent, specific medications have been tested for immune safety in the young.

In the Home

Baby Items

The items used to feed, dress, entertain, transport and sustain a baby all have the potential to be sources of toxic chemicals. This point was driven home recently by the finding of extensive lead-contamination in children's toys that were manufactured outside of the U.S. All items that may come into contact with your baby or are used in preparation for your baby should be scrutinized for chemical safety. Certain plastic items may have the ability to leech endocrine-disrupting chemicals such as bisphenol A and pthalates. Bedding may contain flame retardant chemicals now recognized as potent toxins (such as polybrominated diphenyl ethers). Even some clothing that is brightly colored or has bright colored decorations may contain lead and other harmful toxins. These can build up in your child's body and present immune and other problems.

Chemicals in the Home

As discussed in Chapter 13, homes and apartments can be a major source of hazardous chemicals. These can be found in old paint and solvents deposited from home renovation, household cleaners and insecticides and through mold contamination. Just as was done for the pregnancy, it is important to examine the chemicals in your home and look for opportunities to remove hazardous chemicals. More and more companies are manufacturing cleaners that are "green." It is hoped, but not guaranteed, that they contain fewer toxins and may be useful substitutes.

Smoking in the Home

The dangers from exposure to tobacco smoke continue for the newborn, infant and adolescent just as they did during prenatal development. Environmental tobacco smoke (also called second-hand smoke; see Chapter 16) increases respiratory-based immune inflammation in the child and contributes to a greater risk of asthma, asthma-related hospitalization, and respiratory infections. Beyond the respiratory system there is an increased risk of cardiovascular disease. Exposing your child to tobacco smoke is preventable. For the sake of their child's immune system, parents should seek a smoke-free home and obtain medical support to stop smoking if need be.

Animal Planet

As will be detailed in the chapter on Hygiene and Pets, pets can be a child's best friend. They can also be a friend of your child's immune system. But there appear to be optimum and less optimum times for introducing pets into the household. If the parents themselves are not allergic, then the earlier a furry-type pet appears in your baby's home, the better. Getting a pet for the first time when the child is older actually increases the chances of developing a pet-associated allergy. From the standpoint of the immune system, introducing your baby to the animal planet early on can be a good thing. But do keep in mind these immune-related data are based on large populations of infants and risk of allergies. Your own child could still develop allergies regardless of the timing of getting a pet. This is particularly true if genetic background predisposes a child to allergies.

Hygiene

This is a touchy subject at best because no one would suggest to you that you expose your baby to harmful germs and risk dangerous infections. But the reality is that babies exposed to some occasional bacteria, like those found in barnyard settings, have better and more rapid maturation of their immune systems. Some level of exposure to bacteria or to their cell surface pieces (some of which are also prebiotics) actually help babies to be more prepared immunologically to fight off infections. Additionally, the cost of keeping a 'sterile' household may mean that you are using detergents and cleaning agents with higher concentrations of harmful chemicals. While you completely eliminate bacteria that can help your baby's immune system to mature, you may also be introducing a more dangerous chemical environment into your home.

The bottom line is that you want to protect your baby from the risk of serious infections and to that end sanitation is good. But there is also the possibility of overkill when it comes to sanitation, and in some Western countries we have probably reached that point. Help your baby to stay safe but allow him/her to experience a little bit of the real world as well.

Outside the Home

The Yard, Park, Playground and Sports Fields

Chapter 13 on prenatal strategies provided suggestions for identifying potential risks both outside the house and in the neighborhood. Virtually all outdoor risks considered during pregnancy continue to be a concern during the childhood years. For example, during play children are exposed to the soil surrounding the home and in area parks, school yards, playgrounds and sports fields.

Any prior contamination of these areas with old paint dust, wood preservatives, industrial chemicals or other developmental immune toxins is a concern in the young child. Knowing "where" your child is playing may go beyond a GPS coordinate. Consulting an area historian or past news articles about your town can prove enlightening. Additionally, you might ask local officials if air and soil sampling for toxic chemicals has been conducted recently.

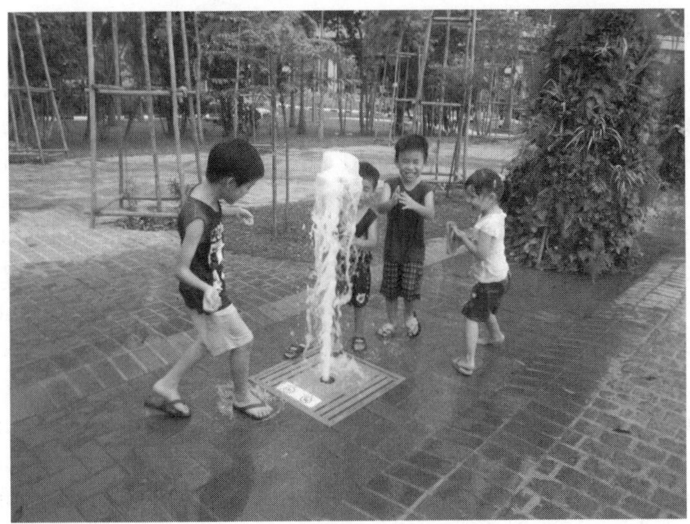

General Surroundings

Exposure to heavy traffic pollution, exhaust particles in the air and pollution-related gases such as sulfur dioxide and ozone are a major concern. The child's airways and breathing patterns are different from those of adults. When placed in the same environment, children are likely to have a higher exposure level to these air pollutants than an adult. For this reason, care as to the air your child breathes is well worth your attention as a parent.

Daycare and Schools

Since a young child is likely to spend a reasonable amount of time in the daycare setting, pre-kindergarten, kindergarten and eventually elementary school, the immune safety of these environments is also on the checklist for parents to consider. Products used for food services, cleaning, lawn care, and building maintenance should be considered just as they would be for your own home. Additionally, air quality is the same issue here for the child as it was for pregnant women in the workplace (see Chapter 16).

Childhood Diet

Just as the diet during pregnancy was important for prenatal immune development and breastfeeding is advantageous for the infant, the child's diet once solid foods are introduced can affect the status of the immune system. In general, those dietary choices that are known to provide health benefits are also supportive of your child's immune system (see Chapter 20). A diet balanced in protein sources with plenty of fruits and vegetables is a good start. Don't forget about the important role of antioxidants (vitamin E, vitamin C, selenium) in immune maintenance and protection against inflammation. Also, continued dietary intake of omega-3 fatty acids is helpful to minimize the negative effects of inflammation. However, your child should be protected against exposure to mercury and PCBs as may occur via contaminated seafood. Remember that childhood obesity and immune-inflammation problems go hand-in-hand. Both need to be prevented and both are influenced dramatically by early life environment and diet. Set your child on a low-inflammation dietary course if possible.

Conclusions

The child's first few years of life represent the second most sensitive period next to prenatal development. Environmental effects on the infant's immune system are capable of determining the level and quality of immune function through later decades of life. Attention to your child's environment including home and property products, the child's diet and the child's surroundings outside the home are all important considerations.

What is the best advice we can provide? Be proactive in molding your child's environment. Know what chemicals your child is being exposed to through bottles, bedding, toys, cleaning agents and your specific home's dust and water. Pay attention to potential risks in daycare, schools, on playgrounds and even on sports fields. You can play an active role in managing your child's immune system for better health. Be proactive in asking your pediatrician the right questions concerning the best timing of vaccinations and drug safety for the developing immune system. Don't be afraid to ask questions or to bring magazine and science articles that help the discussion. By paying attention to your child's environment, you can help his or her immune system to be a supporter and friend for your family's future generation(s).

Overview of Strategies for the Young Child

- The newborn's immune system is relatively immature and needs additional maturation to work effectively.
- The first two to four years of a child's life is a period where parental decisions can have significant and long-lasting impact on the child's immune system and subsequent health risks.
- The strategies provided can serve as a reference guide to avoid immune hazards and promote effective immune development in the young child.

Chapter 15 — Undoing the Damage of the Past in Adulthood

Introduction

After the information we have presented thus far about how the immune system works, what can go wrong, what factors can cause problems and specific strategies for avoiding them, there are bound to be some readers who ask, what do you do when prevention is too late? What if you, a friend or another family member were already exposed to toxins early in life and now have a DIT-related condition? Is suffering the only option? Is there anything that can be done to improve immune health at this point? The answer is yes.

In this chapter, we will go over steps you can take in several areas of your life that, while probably not capable of totally reversing DIT damage, may be able to alleviate symptoms and improve health. The strategies fall into several categories: 1) pharmaceutical medications, 2) food allergies and sensitivities, 3) probiotic intake, 4) natural immune system enhancers, 5) alternative therapies and 6) proven stress reduction techniques. These have all been shown to have a positive impact on the immune system.

Note that whatever course or combination of courses you might consider to alleviate symptoms associated with immune dysfunction, it should be done under the supervision of a physician, complementary integrative medicine MD or alternative healing arts specialist (herbalist, healing work practitioner, etc.). For example, one dose of a natural immune enhancer may be helpful for immune improvement while a higher dose may produce its own harmful side effects. Safety is important whether using a prescription drug or a natural formulation. The information provided in this chapter is designed to serve as a reference for you. Much of the information is taken from a recent review article we prepared for the journal, *Current Medicinal Chemistry*.

Pharmaceutical Medications

Because of the significant number of immune-based diseases and high prevalence of several diseases, pharmaceutical companies have been very active in developing and gaining approval for drugs designed to modulate the immune system. Several of these are based on naturally-occurring chemicals. Others are immune-system derivatives such as cytokines. We will not attempt to list all the drugs here that may be used in immunotherapy as they are extensive in number, rapidly changing and may vary between countries. In fact, the number of immunotherapy drugs currently in the pipeline runs into the hundreds. Pharmaceutical medications offer a significant avenue of therapy under the direction of your physician, but they are not the sole option. Other options that may be considered for addressing immune dysfunction are discussed in the following sections.

Food Allergies and Sensitivities

A sensitivity to foods (specifically proteins found in foods) seems to plague a lot of people who have DIT-related conditions. Sometimes they are outright allergies like an allergy to peanuts that can result in a life-threatening allergic reaction or an allergy to gluten found in wheat and similar grains that is problematic for people with celiac disease. Other times they are just sensitivities that may not show up on allergy tests but can create low-level, chronic inflammation, often throughout the whole body. This chronic, systemic inflammation is a sign of the immune system on hyper-alert status. The problem with this is that the inflammation drains energy from the individual and can even change the ability of the person's body to respond to a viral or bacterial infection.

For instance, research has shown that people with Myalgic Encephalomyelitis/Chronic Fatigue Syndrome (ME/CFS) often have chronic inflammation suggesting that their immune systems are always at work. When ME/CFS patients actually develop an infection, instead of their immune systems revving up further to meet the challenge, their immune systems have a tendency to crash (further discussed in a later chapter). Thus, not only do they not fight off the illness, it may linger in a dormant state within their body to be reactivated later (e.g., herpes viruses).

Diet is something you have some personal control over. If you or someone in your family already has a DIT-related condition, an appointment with an allergist/immunologist is in order. Tests for food allergies can be very revealing. Try avoiding those particular foods for about two months and see if you notice a change. At the end of two months, try adding back in one food at a time and pay close attention to all symptoms in your body (not just those of the DIT-related condition). You may be very surprised by what you notice.

If no allergies are picked up by allergy tests or refraining from eating the suspect foods doesn't make a difference, ask your allergist to help you go on a full-blown elimination diet. This usually requires you to remove all possible allergy-provoking foods (e.g., dairy, wheat, soy, eggs, nuts, etc.) from your diet for a period of time then add them back in one-at-a-time. You would be asked to keep a journal of all reactions and changes in symptoms.

Allergy tests are good, but they only check for changes in IgE levels in the body. Unfortunately, some allergies spike other antibody levels or may be driven by one aspect of T helper cells. Current allergy tests don't check for all possible reactions. That's why a full elimination diet can be more helpful.

While staying away from food allergens can be challenging and not always easy, the benefits can be striking. When your immune system is no longer being geared up for a constant fight, your whole body has a greater chance of relaxing. When a virus or bacterium does strike, your immune system stands a much better chance of fending it off.

Probiotics

Probiotics are getting a lot of attention these days. Turn on the television and it's hard to avoid an ad for probiotic-containing yogurt. Look in the yogurt section of your grocery store, and you'll see yogurt drinks designed to help bolster your immune system. This is because good gut bacteria get destroyed every time you take antibiotics, whenever you're under stress, when you're sick (without needing antibiotics), and by unhealthy diets and lifestyles. However, you need those good gut bacteria both to help you break down food in order to get the nutrients from it and to maintain the health of your intestinal lining. Plus, if you have healthy levels of good gut bacteria, they will overwhelm any harmful bacteria you may encounter. As previously mentioned, they block any spaces for harmful bacteria to get a foothold in your G.I. tract.

This gets to be important if you've ever had your appendix removed. For decades the appendix was thought to be disposable tissue that was prone to infection and could be removed without ill affect. However, in 2008 researchers at Duke University finally discovered exactly what the appendix is intended to do. Apparently, the appendix is where good gut bacteria develop and where extra good bacteria are housed until needed. Without an appendix, you're more vulnerable to infections and to lowered levels of good intestinal bacteria. That's not to say that when your appendix becomes infected, it shouldn't be removed, because once infected it can be life-threatening. However, some appendectomies are done to prevent other infections or make future diagnostics simpler. You and the surgeon should have a long conversation about the necessity of such a procedure.

Natural Immune System Enhancers

In recent years, researchers have begun to identify herbs and fungi (aka mushrooms) that are able to enhance the immune system and/or to restore a more useful immune balance. Even better, they have been able to determine exactly how these substances impact it. We'll include several here in case you're ever interested in trying any. Some could be as simple as adding them to soups, stews, sauces, etc, while others can be taken as teas. Just remember, even though these are "natural" substances, a little goes a long way and at too high a dose, even these can have harmful side effects.

Latin name	Common name	Immune action
Astragalus membranaceus	Milk Vetch Root, Yellow Vetch, Huang qi	— Immune stimulant — Polysaccharides in this plant are capable of enhancing the response to animal vaccines and inducing dendritic cells to mature — Protects against free oxygen radicals
Dichroa febrifuga	Blue Evergreen Hydrangea, Chang shan	— A derivative (halofuginone) has been found to reduce skin collagen and is being considered as a treatment for scleroderma — May treat autoimmune diseases by only suppressing Th17, rather than the entire immune system
Dioscorea alata	Wild Yam, Winged Yam, Water Yam, White Yam	— It can activate both innate and acquired immunity — Elevates serum IgG and IgA levels without impacting IgE
Echinacea purpurea	Purple Coneflower, Black Simpson, Red Sunflower, Comb Flower, Cock up Hat, Missouri Snakeflower, Indian Head and American Coneflower	— Shown to enhance cancer-fighting Th1 activity — Can be consumed as a tea or taken as a capsule
Ganoderma lucidum	Reishi mushroom, Ling chih, Ling zhi, Lucky fungus, Shi uh, "Plant of Immortality"	— Used as an antitumor agent and for its ability to stimulate the immune system — Helps immature dendritic cells mature towards better Th1 immune responses — Reduces oxidative stress in metastatic breast cancer — Inhibits allergic bronchial inflammation — Reduces inflammatory cell migration to the airways
Grifola frondosa	Maitake, Cloud Mushroom	— Has a stimulating effect on the immune system against tumors — Stimulates macrophages — Shifts the balance of T cells toward a Th1 profile (a more mature profile)

(*Continued*)

(Continued)

Latin name	Common name	Immune action
Lentinus edodes	Shiitake, Snake Butter, Pasania fungus, Forest Mushroom, Hua gu	— Increases phagocytotic activities of peripheral macrophages — Ingested orally, they increase the number and ratio of T helper cells — Enhances some vaccine responses — Reduces the negative effects of some inflammatory cytokines during the response to live attenuated vaccines — Elevates cell-mediated immunity including T-dependent immunity against sarcoma
Nigella sativa	Black Seed, Black Cumin, Fitch, "Love in the Mist"	— Triggers apoptotic cell death (programmed cell death that usually doesn't cause inflammation) in colorectal cancer cells — Inhibits allergic airway inflammation
Panax ginseng	Asian ginseng, Chinese ginseng, Korean ginseng, Asiatic ginseng	— Reduces pneumonia-associated lung inflammation and promotes dendritic cell maturation — Protects against stress-induced reduction in Th1 activity — Effective in increasing natural killer cell activity
Phellinus linteus	Sang Hwang, Mesimakobu, Lignum Mushroom	— Extract dissolved in water enhances Th1 cytokine production in a way that reduces allergic responses. — Enhances antibacterial and antitumor function in macrophages
Sophor flavescens Ait	Ku shen, Sophora root	— Several of its constituents scavenge free radicals — Several antioxidants that were isolated increase antiviral immunity against Coxsackie virus B3 — Oxymatrine, an alkaloid from the herb, reduces lung inflammation
Trigonella foeman graecum L	Fenugreek, Greek Hay, Alhova, Bird's Foot, Greek Clover and Hu Lua	— Water-based extracts enhance cell-mediated immune responses and influence the activation of macrophages

Alternative Therapies

Acupuncture

Acupuncture is among the alternative therapies that appears to be capable of producing immunomodulation. As a therapy, acupuncture comes from a thousands-of-years-old Chinese system that involves well-defined lines of energy called meridians. These meridians follow specific paths along the body and at particular points along those lines, different health aspects of the body can be positively affected by the insertion of needles, mild electrical stimulation or pressure. In recent decades, Western science has started to research the ancient claims of health benefits for acupuncture and is finding that some of those claims are valid. One such claim is that acupuncture can help to improve the immune system's function.

According to a study from Japan, acupuncture has the capacity to increase the levels of several immune cytokines. Its ability to do this means that acupuncture may be able to regulate the immune system and help promote better operation in terms of humoral and cell-mediated immunity. Plus, it seems to improve natural killer cell activity as well. In studies that looked at its affects with patients receiving chemotherapy, acupuncture was found to be able to help patients' keep better immune function while under drug treatments that normally suppress the immune system.

Massage Therapy

Massage therapy is another option known to produce immunomodulation. According to an article in the *International Journal of Neuroscience* studies of massage therapy have shown that it is capable of increasing the numbers of natural killer cells in the body and natural killer cell cytotoxicity. And many studies show that massage therapy increases blood circulation and lymph flow while also increasing levels of endorphins (the body's natural pain killers). In its many applications, it shows great benefit for people who receive chemotherapy, surgery or are being treated for significant burns.

Proven Stress Reduction Techniques

Meditation

Meditation is a relaxation technique with thousands of years of practice behind it. While a lot of claims have been made for meditation, Western research is beginning to corroborate those claims particularly in the area of immune system enhancement. One study showed that individuals who meditated produced higher levels of antibodies in response to a flu shot than the control subjects who didn't meditate. What's more, some of the observed biological effects persisted for up to four months beyond the end of the study. There are also studies showing the positive effects that meditation has on the immune systems of people with HIV. In the study, meditation was shown to help people with HIV maintain greater CD4+ T lymphocyte levels. This is important since the CD4+ T lymphocytes are the T helper cells in both Th1 and Th2 categories. The decline in these cells is one of the factors that makes HIV-AIDS so devastating.

Tai Chi

Tai Chi Chuan is an ancient Chinese martial art that is more recently used as a form of exercise. In 2007 the National Institute of Aging and the National Center for Complementary and Alternative Medicine reported on a study of Tai Chi and found that it strengthens the immune system. In one study, it helped senior citizens increase their immunity to shingles, which often occurs in later years as the immune system weakens and is no longer able to hold the varicella zoster (chickenpox) virus at bay. A strengthened immune system was also found to provide greater protection against influenza and other infections in the elderly population.

Conclusions

Immune dysfunction produced through a combination of environmental exposures and the genetic background of the individual can lead to a matrix of increased disease risks. As discussed in a prior chapter, these interlinked immune-related diseases: 1) span a lifetime, 2) involve an increasing percentage of children and adults and 3) negatively impact quality of life. Parts I and II of this book have emphasized both the benefits of preventing immune dysfunction and strategies to boost the odds of achieving that. However, for a large number of older children and adults, the die has already been cast for developmental immunotoxicity and immune-related disease may already be present.

This chapter has provided information for those already experiencing immune dysfunction-associated problems. Some potentially useful medications are already on hand and many new immunomodulating drugs are in the pharmaceutical pipeline. Additionally, there are several alternative approaches that may be helpful either alone or in combination to make changes to the immune system in a way that promotes greater immune balance. Managing current symptoms and minimizing the risk of future immune-based diseases is possible. We encourage you to use this chapter as a reference for consultation with your physician or alternative health professional.

Overview of Undoing the Damage

- Pharmaceuticals offer possible therapies for immune dysfunction. Several exist today and many more will be available in the near future.
- Herbal- and fungal-derived medicinals contain a wealth of immunomodulatory compounds. These are the original source for many drugs and represent a useful immune-correcting option.
- Both prebiotics and probiotics have a role in addressing immune problems.
- Alternative therapies and stress reduction techniques can be excellent adjuncts in strategies to correct immune damage.

Part III — Specific Factors

Chapter 16 — Top 25 Risks

Introduction

Part III of this book provides the often extensive details that led to the suggested strategies we provided in Part II. Though not the lightest reading to be found in this book, the information in Part III explains why we focused on particular strategies earlier. In the present chapter we describe the Top 25 environmental risk factors for your child's immune system. These are the high priority hazards for parents to be aware of. Some proactive strategies to reduce risk were discussed in earlier chapters.

Fortunately, some of the Top 25 risk factors are both important and are also relatively easy to address, such as avoiding tobacco smoke. Others may require more planning and effort (e.g., discussing the timing of childhood vaccinations with pediatricians, minimizing exposure to immunotoxic chemicals in the home and neighborhood). Factors were placed in the Top 25 List based on: 1) how potent the factor was in producing immune damage, 2) how many pregnant women and children were likely to be put in jeopardy, and 3) the quality of the evidence implicating the factor in early life immune impairment. As you might expect, trying to decide which factors came in as #24 and #25 as opposed to which would go in the Appendix was not an easy or precise process. Keep in mind that for certain families, some of those chemicals, drugs and processes listed outside the Top 25 may be considerably more important than some of those in the Top 25.

The Top 25 Concerns

The list of chemicals, mixtures, drugs, physical and psychological factors and conditions described in the following section is intended to help parents and their physicians focus their priorities on the factors of greatest concern. These include chemicals, drugs and conditions that are either well-established as developmental immune health risks or are factors that are suspected as problems based on current research. Additionally, these are factors our babies are likely to be exposed to.

Of course another issue is what lies beyond these 25. There are likely to be many other immune risk factors that have yet to be identified given the very limited amount of DIT safety testing that is currently being performed. The lists we present in this and other chapters are undoubtedly not the whole story. Here are our Top 25 risk factors from top offender to the bottom.

1. *Tobacco Smoke*

The chemicals in tobacco smoke including that of cigarettes can be delivered to the developing baby via the pregnant woman, either by her direct smoking or through passive secondhand smoke. The infant and child may be exposed by others in the household who smoke, and the adolescent could be the one actually doing the smoking. All of these exposures present significant health risks for the developing and immature immune system. The relationship of smoking to both lung cancer and cardiovascular disease in adults has been known for some time. However, a full appreciation for the negative impact of any smoking on the child's immune system is a more recent finding.

Cigarette smoke is not a single chemical. Instead, it is a collection of more than 4,000 chemicals, a significant number of which are potent immunotoxicants and/or carcinogens. The U.S. EPA has a list of more than 90 significant toxicants in tobacco smoke while the list developed by the International Agency for Research on Cancer (IARC) includes more than 80 toxic chemicals. Examples of major toxicants found in cigarette smoke are: hydrogen cyanide, acrolein, formaldehyde, nicotine, lead, styrene, acetaldehyde, benzene, benzo[*a*]pyrene, cadmium, chromium, nitrosamine, tar, acetone, phenol, quinolein, carbon monoxide, cresol and toluene.

Beyond the well-known risk of cancer, why else should you keep your baby's immune system away from any and all cigarette smoke? Recent research has shown that both prenatal and neonatal exposure to cigarette smoke compromises the immune defenses in a baby's airways and increases the likelihood of diseases including asthma, allergies and bronchitis. These diseases are sometimes fatal (e.g., anaphylactic shock) and at a minimum require decades of health management. In addition, they are early-life entryways to additional diseases including behavioral disorders and lung cancer (see Chapter 11).

The oxygen radicals in cigarette smoke damage airway linings making bacterial infections more likely. Additionally, the heavy metals and other chemicals in cigarette smoke skew the baby's immune system toward allergic responses. This significantly increases a baby's risk of asthma and/or respiratory allergies. This combination of toxic effects on the baby's respiratory system can play out in the form of airway vulnerability that lasts for his/her entire life.

But the immune damage does not end there. The same immunotoxicants that elevate Th2 responses and increase the risk of allergic disease also depress immune defenses against viruses and tumor cells. As best as researchers can tell, both the heightened risk of airway disease and allergies as well as the reduced protection against tumors are lifelong changes that may never be corrected. So the damage caused by prenatal, neonatal and juvenile exposure to cigarette smoke has the potential to burden your child with unnecessary and avoidable lifelong chronic disease.

Because exposure to cigarette smoke is largely avoidable and preventable, avoidance of cigarette smoke is priority # 1 in the strategy for protecting your child's immune system.

2. *Alcohol*

Exposure to alcohol represents a serious health risk particularly for the developing baby. Primary exposure occurs through the pregnant and nursing mother but can also occur in infants and older children from certain over-the-counter (OTC) medications that may contain alcohol as a solvent. At higher levels of fetal alcohol exposure, multiple systems are damaged. One group of problematic health outcomes is known as fetal alcohol syndrome (FAS). However, alcohol presents a health risk for the fetus even at lower levels of maternal drinking that may not result in full blown FAS.

Alcohol can disrupt two or more critical windows of immune development. Evidence suggests that early gestational exposure to alcohol causes a change in neurotransmitter receptor expression on immune cells and that change persists into adulthood. This would be expected to alter neuro-immune responses in the offspring. It may be tempting to think that drinking later in the pregnancy, such as in the third trimester, would be less risky than drinking early in the pregnancy. But the third trimester is one of the more sensitive developmental windows for disruption of the immune system by alcohol. In the final trimester of pregnancy, alcohol appears to target immune maturation in the lungs. Alcohol exposure interferes with the interaction between immune cells and lung surfactants. This can create several health problems.

First, it can mean that the defenses in the lungs are not at full capacity in the infant and may have difficulty reaching full capacity even as the child grows. This places the child at a greater risk of airway infections. An additional problem is that the cells involved in inflammatory responses do not mature correctly when exposed to alcohol. They are more likely to produce a hair-trigger response that mis-fires when fighting infections. That means that when they respond during infections, they are far more likely to cause collateral damage to the lungs and other tissues. What happens is that the inflammatory cells overproduce oxygen radicals, and this exhausts an important antioxidant, glutathione. Because antioxidant production is insufficient to prevent damage, the lining of the airways gets damaged by free radicals. This is the collateral damage of concern. Obviously, these types of changes can cause problems not only in the lungs but also in other tissues and organs as the child grows.

What is an immunologically safe level of alcohol exposure for the fetus? Researchers really don't know at present.

3. *Stress*

Stress can take many forms and many environmental, physical and emotional factors can increase stress in pregnant women and directly in young children. Some of these factors are easier for parents to control than others. For example, it may be feasible for parents to avoid dietary-related stress during pregnancy and infancy. However, loss of a family member or a friend is not controllable and could happen quite unexpectedly.

Scientists know that stress linked to bereavement and the mourning process presents a serious challenge for the immune system, and this may be a dilemma some new parents will face. In such cases, the length and intensity of the bereavement-associated stress can influence the problems that may be created for the immune system of both the mother and the unborn child. Knowledge of stressors and their potential impact on the baby's immune system is the starting place for new parents. The immune health goal for parents during pregnancy and in early childhood should be to: 1) identify potential stressors, 2) avoid stress where possible, 3) minimize the intensity of the stress when possible, 4) restrict the stressful period to the shortest duration that is feasible and 5) learn coping strategies and techniques to help get mother and child through the stressful period.

Why does stress deserve such attention? Recent research suggests that in adults, prolonged and/or intense stress can suppress the capacity of our immune system to fight disease. Immune cells respond directly to stress with some cells mobilizing for attack and others taking up defensive positions. This can be useful when fighting infections. However, even in adults, if the stress is too intense or becomes chronic, the overuse of the immune mobilization can lead to an exhausted immune system. In most individuals, the immune system can eventually recover its function if the diseases do not win out (e.g., cancer, pneumonia). However, the situation is different in babies and children. Research has shown that with early-life exposure to significant stress, the baby's and child's immune and neurological systems actually become rewired for different interactions with the environment later in life. This dynamic of sensitivity between the neurological and immune systems is not just a coincidence. Each system is able to influence function in the other. So there are probably more early life imprinted changes that affect both systems in some integrated way than affect just the neurological system or just the immune system alone.

Early, significant periods of stress can imprint on the baby's immune system. This stress permanently alters the way the immune system responds to what would otherwise be considered a normal challenge in the child and the adult. For this reason, prenatal, neonatal and childhood stress has very different health implications compared with stress that adults experience. A 2008 study from Germany found that adult women who had major stress while in the womb had altered immune parameters as adults including elevated blood levels of IL-6. This cytokine is one of the proinflammatory cytokines. Misregulation of IL-6 is often seen in both clinical depression and sleep disorders.

To provide more details, we will discuss different types of stress that can affect the developing immune system.

a) *Psychological stress*

Psychological stress is a real and potent factor in the immune health of children and adults. Recently some scientists have placed psychological stress into a category termed "social toxins." They have suggested that prolonged psychological stress in children can synergize with environmental toxins to damage the child's physiological systems. There is an immune basis for depression in individuals with inflammatory and/or autoimmune disease. Misregulation of those cytokines that promote inflammation, such as IL-6, seems to go hand-in-hand with depression. Alternatively, optimism during times of stress has been shown to reduce inflammation during vaccination responses. This becomes important since the quality and nature of vaccine responses as well as responses to infections will be different based on the mix and levels of cytokines produced.

An example of this can be seen in patients with myalgic encephalomyelitis/chronic fatigue syndrome (ME/CFS). In these patients, the immune system is frequently activated as if they were mounting an inflammatory response to an infection even when they are otherwise well. Baseline levels of IL-6 are usually higher in people with ME/CFS than in people without it. But when the patients are actually fighting an infection, their immune responses can be blunted. The elevated baseline inflammation in ME/CFS patients can actually suppress the needed response against a virus. It is one of the reasons that reactivated herpes viruses are often found in ME/CFS patients. It is also a good example showing that exaggerated immune responses of one type (e.g., inflammation) can actually produce insufficient responses of other needed types (e.g., antiviral protection).

Psychological stress and depression during pregnancy can also result in overproduction of several inflammatory cytokines and mediators including IL-6 and TNF-alpha. This can lead to preterm delivery and additional complications. Stress-promoted inflammation also causes overproduction of oxygen radicals and has been linked to obesity, earlier-life mortality and premature aging of the immune system. Therefore, it becomes very important to interrupt the stress cycle both during pregnancy and childhood.

Parents should recognize that the stress-induced immune vulnerability of children is not restricted only to the prenatal period and infancy. The quality of the childhood environment is important to the status of the immune system and risk of disease. In a study published in 2009 in the Proceedings of the U.S. National Academy of Sciences, the early rearing environment of children (abused or parentally-deprived vs. controls in average households) was found to be related to increased herpes virus reactivation (e.g., mononucleosis, chicken pox, shingles) later in childhood. The researchers proposed that this was due to reduced cell-mediated immune defense against the virus in those children who experienced highly stressful or traumatic events early in life. Other research reported that increased family stress and parental psychiatric symptoms are directly related to immune profiles and herpes virus reactivation among children.

In another recent study of teenage girls and young adult women in western Canada, scientists found that significant interpersonal stress (e.g., think the movie "Mean Girls") sets up the immune system for over-aggressive inflammation when the teenagers had to fight off their next infection. Of note, the effect of the stress on the immune system was not fully apparent until the immune system responded to a disease challenge. Similar findings were reported among adolescent and teenage girls from

French-speaking Canada. Among these girls, an interval of peer group rejection was invariably followed by an interval of increased physical health problems.

These observations all support the fact that childhood stress can set up the immune system for later problems such as the previously mentioned condition, ME/CFS. That condition arises most often in adult women but pediatric cases are increasingly common. Because it can occur in children, early life environmental risk factors appear to be important. Many ME/CFS episodes are triggered either by stress (acute or long term) or by infections where the immune response of the patients is largely inappropriate. Not surprisingly, a high percentage of adults diagnosed with ME/CFS also report childhood trauma in their personal background.

In summary, the relationship between stress and immune status is critically important to your child's health. Ironically, some toxicologists view "stress" as an indirect effect and something to discount in system-specific safety testing. But the developing immune and neurological systems are remarkably sensitive to long term modulation by stress. That fact should be a reminder to us that not all dangers for the developing immune system are from chemicals or drugs.

b) *Physical stress*

Physical stress can also exert an effect on immune cell redistribution throughout the body and on immune function. With low-to-moderate stress such as one might encounter with regular exercise, this can be beneficial in keeping the immune system fine-tuned and ready for action. However, excessive and prolonged physical stress can lead to the same exhausted immune system that is seen with other forms of chronic stress. Extremely rigorous training as may occur with competitive athletes has the potential to reduce antioxidant protection by draining the system of certain micronutrients. Excessive physical stress is known to cause overproduction of several neurological and hormonal factors including the steroid hormone, cortisol. Too high and too prolonged a burst of cortisol will suppress immunity and reduce resistance to disease. While this is a specialized case, over-training can negatively affect several of the body's systems including the immune system.

4. *Traffic Pollution*

According to the U.S. EPA more than 35 million people in the United States live within 300 feet of a major road. Traffic pollution can affect us where we live, commute or work. Exhaust from cars, buses and trucks spew a variety of chemicals into the environment including volatile organic compounds (VOCs) like benzene and 1,3,butadiene, nitrogen dioxides, carbon monoxide, ozone and particulate matter. The particles produced by traffic contain a variety of toxicants, the most serious of which are the polycyclic aromatic hydrocarbons (e.g., benzo[a]pyrene) and metals. Many of these individual chemicals would be on our Top 25 List by themselves. But here are several highly immunotoxic chemicals we have grouped together by virtue of the fact that their emissions result from gasoline- and diesel-engine combustion.

Traffic pollution can contribute to a variety of health problems with many centered on the immune system and can impact the respiratory and cardiovascular systems. This is reflected in a recent study of women in the Seattle, WA area. This study found that women living in proximity to major traffic arteries had reduced natural killer cell activity when compared to women living further away from traffic.

If adult exposure to traffic pollution can damage immune health in the adult, then prenatal and neonatal exposure to traffic pollution appears to be an even more important factor in the immune status of the child. Several recent studies from the US, the UK and Germany indicate that prenatal and early neonatal exposure to traffic pollution increases the risk of childhood asthma and allergies. Exposure to one of the groups of pollutants, polycyclic aromatic hydrocarbons (PAHs), may be particularly important in this risk. A 2009 study in Brazil also found that proximity to the heaviest traffic pollution during pregnancy was an excellent predictor of early neonatal death in the offspring. While this study could not suggest why children were dying at an early age, the immune, respiratory and cardiovascular problems that are associated with early-life, pollutant-induced immunotoxicity may play some role.

Parents may not be able to easily control whether their child lives far away from heavy traffic. But in these circumstances, there may be ways to improve the air quality within the home and minimize exposure as much as is possible. Efforts to minimize exposure of pregnant women and young children to heavy traffic pollution should pay dividends in reduced risk of chronic disease.

5. *Lead*

Lead is a naturally-occurring heavy metal that has had extensive commercial use for a lengthy period of human history. In fact, unlike gold or silver, lead was the metal of the masses in many ancient civilizations. It was so common in the tableware of ancient Rome and tainted so much of the food consumed by Rome's leaders, that it is thought to have played a role in the downfall of the Roman Empire. Even then, acute lead poisoning was known. But the many health problems created by prolonged exposure to lower levels of lead were not recognized until centuries later.

Lead exposure affects children worldwide with much of the exposure linked to lead that was previously deposited in the environment. During recent decades, a major public health effort has led to the reduction of lead used in gasoline and paints in the United States and many other counties. However, some countries still use lead in gasoline. Additionally, lead can still be found in several household products (e.g., brunette hair dyes and red lipsticks). Today, the global economy means that lead exposure may come from surprising and unexpected sources. For example, the discovery that many toys imported into the U.S. from China contained significant amounts of lead brought home a new reality for parents. Local standards for lead do not always translate into the same level of protection for our children. Given the globalization of trade, immunological and neurological safety can sometimes reflect the lowest safety standard across the globe.

Apart from new and unexpected sources of lead, the health impact of lead already present in the environment is significant. Deteriorating paint and dust from older housing contributes significantly to the exposure of children. However, depending upon their job, parents may be exposed occupationally as well. Most of the attention with lead toxicity has been focused on neurological affects (e.g., IQ deficits and behavior changes in children). However, the developing immune and neurological systems appear to be similar in their sensitivity to lead. Lead has the capacity to infiltrate most tissues and to inappropriately substitute itself for other physiological components (e.g., zinc which is needed for brain development, calcium which is needed for bone growth). When it does this, it causes disruption of the original function within the body (e.g., enzyme action). With lead-induced DIT, relatively minor physiological alterations can produce major changes in the immune system of the offspring.

Lead exposure can affect virtually all sectors of the immune system. Macrophages are targeted by lead, and this can result in inappropriate inflammatory responses (e.g., overproduction of free radicals). Production of antibodies is altered by lead such that preference is given toward production of IgE antibodies. These are the antibodies that cause mast cells to release histamine during allergic reactions. For this reason lead exposure is likely to contribute to childhood allergic disease. Additionally, changes in T cell function caused by lead appear to create a predisposition for autoimmune reactions. Lead exposure can also cause a reduction in cell-mediated immunity (CMI). The reduced CMI response capacity raises concern regarding the protection of the child against viruses and tumor cells. The exact combination of these changes that may occur in a given individual appears to depend in part on the developmental stage during which the baby is exposed, the level of the exposure and the sex of the baby.

In the 1970s lead exposures that produced an accumulation below ten micrograms per deciliter of blood were thought to be safe in children. We now know that even lower levels of lead produce neurological deficits and are likely to produce immune problems as well. Therefore, lead is an important contaminant to avoid across all stages of a child's life.

6. *Mercury*

Like lead, mercury is a naturally-occurring metal that has been mined since ancient times. Ironically, the recent move to "greener" energy-efficient fluorescent light bulbs that contain mercury has caused some previously closed mercury mines to be reopened in certain countries in order to produce enough mercury to make these types of light bulbs. In this case, "green" may mean sicker for some children.

Mercury has a long history of use among ancient civilizations, in ointments and cosmetics and later in alchemy. During the 18th and 19th centuries it was employed in the making of felt hats. Because exposure to mercury at sufficient levels produces progressive neurological/psychological problems, the phrase "mad as a hatter" was an appropriate description of the health risks in the felt hat-producing industry. This probably inspired the Mad Hatter character in *Alice in Wonderland.*

The same could have been said of those involved in the early silver-plating industry around 1,800 in Britain. Because of mercury vapor released in the early plating process for making tableware, many of those craftsmen spent their later years in insane asylums. As with lead, the health effects of high levels of exposure have been known for a considerable time. But the insidious health effects of lower levels of exposure were only recently identified.

Mercury use was extensive during the 20th century and continues even today. During the 20th century it was included in common disinfectants. It remains a fixture of dental amalgams and, until recently, was still produced in thermometers. It is a component of some medicinals in western countries and Asia appearing in some over-the-counter medicines such as laxatives, diaper rash ointments, eye drops and contact lens fluids. It has also been used as a preservative in some vaccines (as Thimeresol). As previously mentioned, one of the current health controversies concerns its presence in the new energy efficient fluorescent light bulbs. The question one would have to ask is, does it make sense to remove the mercury from vaccines only to bring more of it into our homes through government-mandated lighting? If the bulb breaks, are you prepared for a toxic clean up?

Because mercury is a persistent environmental metal, it, like PCBs, which are discussed later, can bio-accumulate in the food chain. For example, larger fish that feed on smaller fish exposed to mercury can accumulate a very high level of mercury in their tissues well beyond the levels of mercury found in their local bodies of water. As a result, fish like tuna and salmon are a significant health concern particularly when eaten by pregnant women.

Mercury can affect multiple physiological systems. In addition to the immune and neurological systems, the gastrointestinal tract, cardiovascular system and kidneys are at risk. Immune effects linked with early life exposure include a higher risk of autoimmune responses such as those found in lupus, allergic reactions and excessive tissue damage from inflammatory reactions including the overproduction and misdirected action of oxygen radicals and peroxynitrite (one of the free radical molecules that is formed when oxygen radicals and nitric oxide interact). In fact, it is likely that the cardiovascular health risks are linked, in part, to the immune-inflammation problems and overproduction of oxygen radicals. Because of the extreme sensitivity of the baby's immune and neurological systems to mercury, it is a major environmental factor of concern for the child.

7. *Dioxin*

Dioxins are among the most extensively studied classes of toxic chemicals in our environment. In reality there are tens to hundreds of chemical forms that fall under the general name, "dioxin." But the most toxic of these is abbreviated as TCDD since its chemical name is 2,3,7,8-tetrachlorodibenzo-p-dioxin. Because it is the most toxic and of greatest health concern, most other forms of dioxins are compared against TCDD to determine their level of toxicity. If you are reading about such chemicals, you may encounter the designation TCDD most often. We will use this in our discussions.

TCDD is known to cause immune, reproductive and other developmental problems at low levels of exposure. The fetus can receive dioxins across the placenta, and they are also passed to the infant through breast milk. TCDD and other dioxins are fat-loving (called lipophilic) chemicals, which can be stored in the fat of the mother or the child for decades.

TCDD is produced as a waste product of numerous industrial activities such as backyard-burning and commercial incineration particularly of plastics, paper and pulp production and paper bleaching. While EPA regulations and industrial changes have made an impact in reducing dioxin output, there is still a significant amount present in our environment considering its extreme toxicity. TCDD was one of the chemicals found in the defoliant, Agent Orange, and was involved in the Niagara Falls, NY, Seveso, Italy and Times Beach, MO contaminations.

While TCDD and other dioxins are in the environment, the majority of our exposure comes through the food we eat, in particular meat, dairy and fish. For example, a 2001 study showed that farm-raised freshwater fish and butter are prominent sources of TCDD and other dioxins, and the FDA has recommended that fish with TCDD concentrations above 50 parts per trillion not be eaten.

Knowledge that very low levels of TCDD affects the developing immune system has been around since the 1970s. Early studies in rodents showed that exposure to dioxin during gestation caused the thymus gland to atrophy prematurely in the offspring. Not surprisingly, this resulted in changes in T cell function and the suppression of certain immune functions. This immunosuppression produces an increased susceptibility to some infections. But only in the last three years has the broader range of DIT effects caused by exposure to TCDD become clear.

Early-life exposure to TCDD actually disrupts the entire network of T cell development and also affects other immune cells. Because of this, susceptibility to certain infections may be one of the first immunotoxic effects seen. However, it turns out that, while TCDD causes a deficiency of some T cells that we need to develop, it also causes the thymus to release some cells that never should have been allowed out of the thymus because they cause reactions to our own bodies. Additionally, TCDD interferes with a second level of protection against self-reactions that involve our regulatory T cells. This means that in later life, the risk of autoimmunity appears to be increased. So paradoxically, both increased risk of infections and harmful autoimmune responses can occur, meaning that the immune system can't fight off harmful invaders but attacks its own body with a vengeance.

A final problem caused by in utero exposure to TCDD is the misregulation of inflammatory responses. When the immune system is responding to an infection such as influenza, macrophages and other cells work hard to clear the virus while minimizing collateral damage to the airways. In one model study, exposure to TCDD in utero with later exposure to influenza virus, led to difficulty removing the virus from the lungs and damaged the airways due to excessive inflammation. This outcome causes a higher risk of: 1) immediate death from influenza or 2) additional health problems such as a higher risk of secondary bacterial pneumonia.

Beyond that, damage to lung epithelia and excessive oxygen radical production would be expected to increase the risk of adult lung disease including cancer. For this reason, exposure to TCDD produces a triple whammy for the developing immune system: short term increased risk of certain infections, longer term risk of autoimmunity and increased risk of inflammatory-associated conditions that can lead to cancer.

8. *Polychlorinated Biphenyls (PCBs)*

Like the dioxins, polychlorinated biphenyls (PCBs) come in approximately 100–200 forms (called PCB congeners). In fact, in the environment, it is more common to find mixtures of PCBs than to find any single form. This is because most industrial applications of PCBs used mixtures rather than one purified congener. Single PCB forms are found more often in research laboratories.

PCBs were used in a wide range of industrial applications from the 1930s to the early 1970s. They were considered a chemical of exceptional utility that drove much of the developed world's industrial progress. PCBs were employed in transformers and capacitors, coolants and lubricators, in coatings for electric wiring, caulking, adhesives, wood floor sealants, paint, carbonless paper for copying, and hydraulic fluids. In fact, they were so important that many companies (Westinghouse, Monsanto, General Electric, Bayer) gave their own particular mixtures of PCBs specialized trade names.

By the 1970s, their health risks were becoming apparent and PCB production was eliminated for some products. However, they continued to be used in transformers and their release into the environment remained a concern. Additionally, because PCBs persist for prolonged periods of time, their heavy industrial use meant that environmental contamination was already significant. For example, earlier industrial production by companies like General Electric led to river sediment contamination (e.g., the Hudson River) that is still an issue today. Given their persistence, the use of PCBs in prior decades continues to present a major health concern particularly for our children. In fact, most of the advisories against eating fish from certain bodies of water are based on either PCB or mercury concentrations.

The appropriate public response to PCB contamination has been a contentious issue over the decades. This was reflected by an event in 1981 involving the then Governor of New York State and the tallest building in Binghamton, NY, an 18-story building at 44 Hawley St. occupied largely by state government offices. In February 1981 the building was contaminated by significant amounts of PCBs as well as lesser amounts of other toxicants. This occurred when, during a fire, a transformer cracked under extreme heat, and the resulting electrical fire spread PCB-contaminated soot throughout the building. The soot had entered every nook and cranny of the offices and was even found in closed file cabinets. Local health officials were worried. But even as cleanup began via starts and stops, the then governor of New York State, Hugh Carey, seemed unconcerned by the health risks proclaiming he would "here and now walk into Binghamton in any part of that building, and swallow an entire glass of PCBs and then run a mile afterwards."

We are fortunate that today's mothers do not have to follow that state executive's guide to better health. Ironically, some short term health studies were conducted on local employees who had been allowed to enter the building to remove personal items not long after the fire. But while the more significant concern for their personal health would have played out over a much longer period of time, the even greater issue would have concerned the health of children later born to exposed female employees.

Today PCB exposure occurs largely through eating contaminated fish, drinking contaminated water, breathing air around contaminated sites (e.g., Superfund sites, landfills), and operating old electrical appliances. The reason that eating contaminated fish is such a concern involves both the persistence of PCBs in body fat and the increasing accumulation of PCBs as one moves up the food chain. Thus, large fish that feed on other aquatic animals can have accumulated PCB concentrations that may be a thousand fold greater than the PCB levels of the water in which they live.

At higher levels, PCB exposure can produce skin rashes and acne. But in the young, exposures at lower levels produce an elevated risk of immune and reproductive problems. The following examples were introduced earlier in the discussion of diseases. In a Denmark and Harvard University study, researchers examined mother–child pairs in the Faroe Islands who consumed a largely marine diet. They measured the relationship between PCB levels in the body of the mothers and seven-year-old children and the ability of the children to respond immunologically to childhood vaccinations (DPT). They found that the higher the level of PCBs in the children, the poorer their response to the vaccinations. However, of all the measurements taken at different ages, the best indicator of the antibody response to the vaccine in the seven-year-old child was the level of the PCBs that were present in the cord blood when that child was born. This is important because it suggests that the damage to the immune system that impacted the later vaccine response probably happened during the pregnancy. The effect was significant since 28% of the children had such a poor immune response to the vaccinations that they were unlikely to be protected against an infection.

Similar findings have been seen with PCB exposure among the Inuits in Canada. In this population exposed to PCBs and other toxicants, ear infections were more common than expected during the first year of life. Recurrent ear infections were also more common among Dutch school children who had been exposed to PCBs. The cumulative studies suggest that early life exposure to PCBs carries a substantial risk for increased incidence of infant infections, requires an increased use of antibiotics and reduces the protection from diseases that vaccinations usually provide children.

The fact that significant prenatal exposure to PCBs is likely to cause increased childhood infections carries a second link to health risk. If serious bacterial infections occur in the newborn, there is likely to be a need for the use of antibiotics. Use of antibiotics in the newborn also carries its own risk for later immune dysfunction and health problems in the child. This will be discussed in a subsequent section, but the reality is that exposure to PCBs can start a vicious cycle. PCBs can impair the developing immune system resulting in more neonatal infections. This in turn may lead to heavy use of antibiotics. The antibiotic use can produce further immune system alterations in the child that, in turn, increases the risk of additional diseases.

9. *Steroid Drugs*

Steroids are most widely known for the sex-related steroids, including the testosterone-like muscle building drugs (anabolic steroids) illegally used by some professional athletes, and the drugs used for suppressing inflammation and treating both allergic and autoimmune diseases (glucocorticoids). Steroids are representative of a wide category of natural and synthetic fat-loving chemicals including sex and adrenal hormones, digitalis and vitamin D. Cholesterol is a main component of steroid hormones in the body.

Steroidal compounds are used for a variety of human health and physiological considerations. Many steroidal drugs are anti-inflammatory and are used to treat autoimmune and inflammatory diseases. An example of a potent drug used for this purpose is the corticosteroid, prednisone, which is used to treat diseases such as rheumatoid arthritis. Dexamethasone and betamethasone are also steroid drugs used in various medical treatments. Because glucocorticoids are immunosuppressive, their use in otherwise healthy individuals can cause an increased risk of infections and other diseases. The risk to the child is even greater since dose sensitivity and the range of effects appear to be greater in the young when compared to adults. Corticosteroid therapy used for fetal lung maturation has been reported by some research groups to contribute to an elevated risk of childhood asthma.

Anabolic steroids used in body building are based on testosterone derivatives. They can produce numerous adverse effects that impact reproductive organs and behavior. However, the immune system is also impacted. Significant and/or prolonged use of these steroids will also suppress natural killer cell activity and antibody production.

Early life exposure to other sex steroids can be harmful for the immune system. Diethylstilbesterol (DES) is a synthetic estrogen that is a known human carcinogen. It was used during the 1940–70s to prevent miscarriage. However, female babies exposed in utero had an elevated risk of developing reproductive problems and certain cancers as adults. There was evidence pointing toward the capacity of prenatal DES exposure to produce immune abnormalities including an elevated risk of autoimmune disease. Not surprisingly for endocrine disrupting chemicals, exact health risks can differ based on the sex of the baby. Some studies suggest that prenatal DES exposure changes the entire wiring of the immune system. This rewiring means that interactions between the environment and the adult immune systems are often abnormal and unpredictable. As is the case with most endocrine disrupting chemicals (EDCs), parents need to be diligent to protect their children from potentially harmful EDC exposure.

10. *Bisphenol A*

Bisphenol A is an endocrine disruptor and is an important component of many polycarbonate plastic compounds and plastic derivatives including epoxy resins. Bisphenol A can be found in various plastic products. It has also been reported in the plastic linings of some cans containing fruits, vegetables and sodas. Polycarbonate plastic is clear, almost shatter-proof and is used in many products including baby bottles. The toxicity concern is that bisphenol A can leach out of plastics and enter the body. Using plastic containers in the microwave, putting them in the dishwasher and exposing the plastics to harsh detergents can increase the leaching of bisphenol A from these products.

In the body, bisphenol A can act like estrogen and disrupt endocrine balance. Based on model studies, the primary effects of prenatal exposure to bisphenol A are on the immune, neurological, and hormone-influenced (breast, prostate) tissues. In human studies, higher bisphenol A levels have been associated with an increased risk of cardiovascular disease and diabetes. These findings make biological sense based on what is known about bisphenol A. Many governments and federal agencies are currently evaluating their course of action in potentially restricting exposure of children to bisphenol A, and Canada has already banned its use in baby bottles. In the meantime, parents can be prudent by examining plastics carefully. Bisphenol A is found in some Type 3 and Type 7 plastics, identified by the number 3 or 7 inside a triangle on the bottom of plastic products.

11. *Cocaine*

Cocaine in various forms is among the drugs of abuse that cause the greatest concern for the developing fetus and newborn. Cocaine abuse is known to impair immune function and decrease resistance to infectious agents. For example, it is a major factor influencing the extent of viral spread after HIV infection and as a result, facilitating the development of full blown AIDS. Exposure in utero via the mother has been reported to depress both the number of CD4+ T lymphocytes needed to promote most antigen responses and to suppress T lymphocyte responses. For this reason, it is an obvious, potent and avoidable risk factor for the immune system of the developing child.

12. *Marijuana*

Marijuana, also known formally as *Cannabis sativa,* is the most commonly used illicit drug in many Western countries. Use by both teenagers and pregnant women is a significant concern for the developing immune system well as the developing neurological system. The active compound in marijuana is a psychoactive cannabinoid. It interacts with specialized cannabinoid receptors on cells in the body. Activation of these receptors, such as the cannabinoid receptor type 2, can produce profound effects on immune function. Additionally, these receptors play an important role in organ formation during prenatal development where they interact with the endogenous cannabinoid our own body produces. Not surprisingly, exposure to improper amounts of cannabinoid during critical windows of a child's development can impact both brain and immune development.

A recent study found that prenatal exposure to marijuana via the pregnant mother impaired intellectual development among school age children. The exact deficits that occurred were related to the timing of marijuana use by the mother (e.g., first vs. second trimester). Prenatal exposure to marijuana also predicts a higher rate of marijuana use by the adolescent-teen offspring. This is during a period when important neurological maturation is occurring in the child.

Marijuana use in adults can produce immunosuppression with dampened inflammatory responses. In healthy individuals, it can reduce resistance to infectious agents, and it can present an added health risk. However, because they are immunosuppressive, cannabinoid extracts may have a role in treating some autoimmune and inflammatory diseases much like steroid drugs.

Prenatal and lactational exposure to marijuana has been reported to decrease the ratio of T helper cells to T cytotoxic lymphocytes and to blunt T cell responses. While cannabinoids may have a therapeutic role in chronic inflammatory disease, they represent a significant hazard for the normal development of the immune system. At least in outcome, prenatal and lactational exposure of babies to marijuana is similar to exposing babies to glucocorticoid steroids.

13. *Overuse/Early Use of Antibiotics*

Antibiotics are among the miracle drugs of the 20th century. They have saved countless human lives from severe bacterial infections such as typhoid, cholera, tuberculosis, staphylococcus and streptococcus bacteria. They also protect our pets from life threatening diseases. There are numerous medical reasons why pregnant women and newborns may need to use antibiotics. That is a medical decision between the doctor and parents.

However, the use of antibiotics in the newborn appears to carry previously unrecognized health risks that may be appropriate to discuss with pediatricians when treatment options are considered. Recent studies suggest that antibiotic use during the baby's first year may elevate the risk of childhood asthma. This risk is further increased as more rounds of antibiotics are needed for the infant.

Risk of immune problems appears to be increased. Immune risk associated with prenatal exposure to antibiotics. Use of antibiotics by the mother during pregnancy was found to cause an increased risk of childhood asthma in one study. In a second study conducted in Europe, maternal use of antibiotics during pregnancy increased the risk of both allergies (rhinitis and eczema) as well as wheeze in the infant. The exact reason why the antibiotics produce this effect is not known.

14. *Trichloroethylene (TCE)*

Trichloroethylene is a chlorinated hydrocarbon that has been used extensively as an industrial solvent. The most common uses for TCEs were in the dry cleaning industry and across manufacturing industries where it was used as a degreaser for metal parts of machinery. Because of this widespread use, TCE is found in many hazardous waste sites. It is a contaminant of the soil and groundwater surrounding these sites. Examples of TCE contaminated water can be found across the United States (e.g., Endicott, NY; Dayton, OH; Camp Lejune, NC; Salina, KS; Vero Beach, FL; Tucson, AZ).

Federal and state agencies have differed on their regulations concerning the health risk of TCE. However, its use in industry and by the military has gradually decreased in recent years. Yet, the contamination from prior use is the present concern for the exposure of children.

Significant evidence suggests that TCE exposure can alter immune function. In particular, adult exposure to TCE is thought to promote autoimmune disease and to exacerbate the condition where it may preexist. In model studies, prenatal exposure was found to alter T cell development, increase the risk of damage by oxygen radicals and alter neurobehavioral development as well. Research suggests that early-life exposure to TCE presents a likely risk of immune dysfunction in children. Therefore, the exposure of babies and children to this contaminant of soil and water should be a concern for parents.

15. *Nonylphenol*

Nonylphenol is an organic chemical termed a non-ionic surfactant (meaning it can form a detergent-like coating). It is used in the production of detergents, wood and metal products, pesticides and spermacides in contraceptives. Additionally, its derivatives can be found as air pollutants released during wastewater treatment. Nonylphenol is included in this section because this organic chemical acts as an environmental estrogen. Its use was recently restricted by the European Union because of health concerns. However, it can still be found in some household products in the U.S. including commercial and household cleaning products, arts and craft products with epoxy resins and some products used in home maintenance.

Because of its estrogenic activity, nonylphenol was among five endocrine disruptors that were recently evaluated by the U.S. National Toxicology Program (NTP). That evaluation found that nonylphenol was a potent developmental immunomodulator. In model studies exposure to nonylphenol produced immunotoxic changes in the offspring that were not seen in adults exposed to similar doses. Among the changes seen were toxicity to macrophage- and granulocyte-type cells and increases in natural killer cell activity. Some of the changes differed according to the sex of the offspring. These findings suggest that significant caution should be taken to avoid exposing pregnant women or babies to this chemical or its by-products.

16. *Perfluorooctanoic Acid (PFOA)*

PFOA is a fluorinated compound that also goes under the name of C8. It is used in both industrial and commercial applications and is a commonly encountered contaminant in our environment. It is known to modify lipid components of cells affecting the immune system, the liver and the reproductive system. It is also a carcinogen. PFOA is present in microwaveable popcorn bags, Teflon, some food wrapping, stain-resistant carpets, clothes, furniture and industrial waste. It has been an important component of most non-stick or chemical-resistant household products and was previously hailed as a virtual miracle chemical of the 20th century because of its ability to protect surfaces from stains. But we now know that the luxury and the convenience of having these products may have come at a price. PFOA is now considered as a dangerous toxin that is distributed widely in our environment.

Exposure can occur via contaminated drinking water, food, and through dust in air. Use of Teflon-coated cookware can contribute to exposure. Like PCBs, PFOA persists for a long time in the environment.

Adult human studies were conducted in 2005–2006 among Ohio and West Virginia communities in what became known as the C8 project. These communities were located in an area where C8 had been produced for decades and had been exposed to the chemical through their drinking water. Blood samples were taken and analysis performed on more than 50,000 people in this study. Higher amounts of PFOA exposure were associated with reduced levels of the antibody, IgA. This antibody is important in the protection of the eye, gut and other mucosal areas of the body. Additionally, a marker of potential risk of autoimmunity, anti-nuclear antibodies, was elevated in association with higher C8 exposure. This type of change can reflect an increased risk of autoimmune diseases such as lupus. Model studies also support the human immune results. PFOA was found to exert profound effects on the immune system by causing: 1) the thymus to atrophy, 2) T cell populations to change and 3) antibody response to be reduced.

At least some prenatal exposure is likely for most babies. In a recent study at the John's Hopkins School of Public Health, PFOA was detected in 100% of 299 cord blood samples tested. The question then becomes when is that exposure sufficient to be a health problem?

17. *Arsenic*

Arsenic is a common, naturally-occurring metal found in the earth's crust. It is often found in sulfur, silver and gold-containing ores. It has long been known to be a potent poison. Occupational exposure was primarily focused on those working with industrial and agricultural wastes. Most environmental exposures occur from: 1) drinking water taken from areas where the sediment is high in arsenic, 2) from areas surrounding hazardous waste sites or 3) from wood products treated with arsenic-containing preservatives. One of the more recent concerns was the finding that many pieces of playground equipment for children included preserved wood contaminated with arsenic.

Arsenic exposure can affect many systems since it disrupts normal cellular metabolism and energy production causing cells to die. At high levels of exposure, this can lead to functional failure in many different organs. For the immune system, arsenic exposure produces increased oxidative stress and increased production of cytokines that support inflammation. Exposure of children is a concern as discussed by Dr. MaryJane Selgrade, an immunotoxicologist with the U.S. EPA, in a recent report. In utero exposure to arsenic is associated with immunosuppression as well as a concern for increased risk of allergies. So parents should pay attention to potential sources of arsenic (e.g., in drinking water and on playgrounds) in their child's environment.

18. *Genistein*

Genistein is an isoflavone and a major phytoestrogen found in soy and soy-based products such as soy-based infant formulas. As such, genistein competes with estrogen in our own bodies for binding to the estrogen receptor(s). It affects the immune system because many immune cells have the estrogen receptor. Exposure is usually through diet.

The overall role of genistein in health is not a simple story and appears to be partly age- and sex-dependent. In some studies in adults, genistein has been reported to produce beneficial anti-inflammatory and antitumor effects. This is likely due to its capacity to greatly alter cytokine production. But parents need to remember that the immunomodulatory effects seen in adults with immune-based disease are probably not helpful for the proper development of an otherwise healthy immune system.

Most studies agree that babies and children are extremely sensitive to genistein when compared to adults. In model studies, gestational exposure to genistein seemed to target gene expression in the thymus as well as natural killer cells. It also altered antibody production. Additionally, activity of T regulatory cells was affected by early-life exposure to genistein. But the outcomes differed depending on the sex of the offspring.

Given the sensitivity of the baby's system to genistein and the fact that it can alter gene expression in the developing thymus, parents need to pay attention to potential exposure. Excessive and prolonged exposure to estrogen-like substances such as genistein may skew the immune responses in children and cause increased susceptibility to some diseases. However, female and male children are likely to differ with respect to specific adverse health risks. Recently, a 2008 National Toxicology Program report based on model studies suggested that early-life exposure to significant levels of genistein may present an elevated risk for some cancers in females.

The age at which a child is exposed to genistein and how much he/she is given (or are exposed to in the case of prenatal exposure) seems to be most important. A recent study in humans suggested that genistein intake by adolescent women was associated with a slight reduction in breast cancer rate. However, the effect was not seen following either fetal exposure or later life exposure to genistein.

19. *Atrazine*

Atrazine is an herbicide used to kill broadleaf and grassy weeds in crops such as corn, sugar cane, sorghum and evergreen trees. It is one of the most widely used herbicides in the United States and is among a group of herbicides and pesticides that has been reported to possess endocrine-disrupting activity. In the United States alone, more than 75 million pounds of atrazine are produced each year. In its pure form, it is a white, odorless powder.

Atrazine is applied to agricultural fields and is also used near highways and railways to kill weeds. It can be sprayed onto fields either before crops start growing or after they have emerged from the ground. The chemical is very slow to break down after it is applied to soils, so it can enter both ground and surface water. With agricultural use, it takes about one year to degrade half of the concentration of atrazine in soil. Atrazine can occur on dust particles and is usually found in higher concentrations near superfund sites as well. Wells used for drinking water can be contaminated with atrazine, and it is found at lower levels in the drinking supplies of many cities. Exposure of pregnant women and children would largely occur through: drinking water, contact with contaminated dirt, living near agricultural fields that are sprayed or living near contaminated superfund sites.

Atrazine is thought to interfere with hypothalamus-pituitary regulated sex hormones such as prolactin, and this would be a major concern particularly during development. Among atrazine's reported effects in adults is that it can disrupt ovulatory cycling by inhibiting the surge of luteinizing hormone and prolactin. Following prenatal exposure to atrazine, there is a reported delay in mammary gland development.

For the developing immune system, model studies found that prenatal and lactational exposure to atrazine produced alterations of the immune system at several ages after birth. Males and females differed in the extent and nature of their immune changes. For example, males exhibited elevated immune responses as juveniles but these effects were not present in adult males. In contrast, females had no marked immune changes as juveniles but showed suppressed immune function as adults.

20. *Cadmium*

Cadmium is a naturally occurring metal that is found in zinc, iron, and lead ores. It is also released during volcanic eruptions and forest fires. The most common uses of cadmium are in nickel-cadmium rechargeable batteries, pigments in electronics, and coatings and stabilizers of plastic products. A major source of exposure to cadmium is via tobacco smoke (a potent cause of DIT), but exposure can also result from fossil fuel combustion, waste incineration, mining operations, phosphate fertilizer application and emissions from hazardous waste sites. For children, the more likely sources of exposure include: 1) eating some foodstuffs, 2) parental smoking and 3) air near hazardous waste/industrial sites. Most of the intake from foods comes from crops grown in cadmium-rich soil or meat from animals which have eaten cadmium-containing plants.

At higher levels of exposure and chronic moderate exposure in adults, cadmium is known to damage the immune system. Effects include decreased antibody production, cell-mediated immunity and resistance to infectious disease. Cadmium damages the thymus and increases the incidence of a process known as apoptosis (programmed cell death). Inflammatory cells such as macrophages are also affected and can respond by overproducing oxygen and nitrogen free radicals. Excessive oxidative damage results, and there is a depletion of the protective antioxidative factor, glutathione.

When glutathione is depleted, cells and tissues are left vulnerable to damage by free radicals. The damage can take the form of DNA mutations, cell surface damage (e.g., lipid peroxidation) and cell death. Oxidative damage also increases the risk of heart disease. However, data for early-life, lower-level exposure of the immune system to cadmium are limited. In one study in eastern Germany during the 1990s, higher urinary cadmium levels in school children were reported to be associated with immune suppression.

Based on the data that are available and the known role of cigarette smoke in DIT, cadmium is a pollutant worthy of parental concern.

21. *Nickel*

Nickel is a common metal that is used to produce alloys. It is naturally occurring, is deposited in soils and sediment and is released into the air and water. It is a common environmental component of several metallurgical practices and is found in inexpensive jewelry, orthodontic appliances as well as nickel-cadmium batteries. The metal can serve as a potent allergen by forming complexes with proteins in one's own body to produce "new antigens." The immune system will recognize and respond to these "new antigens." This often results in allergic dermatitis when nickel comes into contact with the skin. Recent studies suggest that exposure to nickel can change the expression of a number of genes involved with the immune system. Many of the effects are seen in dendritic cells and involve the way in which antigen is presented to T lymphocytes (see Chapter 4). Inhaled nickel can also produce adverse affects for the immune system. Depending upon the level and duration of exposure, the effects can include decreased lung function, asthma, bronchitis, lung cancer and nasal cancer. However, the latter two effects are most commonly a result of occupational exposure to nickel.

The data suggest that parents should be cautious about exposing their children to nickel. The major risk is the possibility of an allergic hypersensitivity response.

22. *Mold-Derived Toxins*

Unlike some of the other toxins in this Top 25 list, mold-derived toxins or mycotoxins are not synthetic but occur in nature during the normal growth of certain species of molds. In fact, if a family is trying to avoid pesticide-laden food and is replacing it with organic produce, mycotoxins would be one of the potential concerns that should be avoided. They are a potential hazard for the child's immune system, and exposure occurs via both food and air. While the health risks of food contaminants like the grain storage toxin, aflatoxin, have been known for some time, concerns about the potential dangers of airborn toxins produced by "black mold" are more recent.

a) *Black mold — Stachybotrys chartarum*

Toxins from black mold often found in basements and damp areas in homes and buildings appear to cause inflammation in the airways and brain, including possible neurological symptoms. Contamination of household products, toys and outdoor soil with mold toxins are one of the major concerns for the childhood home, daycare and school environment. Molds such as black mold can grow on fiberboard, gypsum board, wallpaper, insulation materials, drywall, carpet, fabric and upholstery.

Many mold toxins are both immunotoxic and neurotoxic. The effects of problematic exposures seem to range from suppression of some immune responses and higher risk of infections to an increased likelihood of respiratory allergies (causing some individuals who were previously unaffected to develop allergies against non-mold allergens). Mold toxins can also increase the risk of airway infections contributing to chronic sinusitis.

Most of the exposure to these toxins is through the air we breathe in indoor areas with mold growth. Exposure to these molds can: 1) damage the airway system, 2) increase the risk of allergy symptoms and 3) dampen the sense of smell. As with any toxin, some are more potent than others, and the dose and exposure route can matter. One of the most potent immunotoxic drugs known and one used for organ transplants, cyclosporin A, was derived from molds.

b) *Mycotoxins as food contaminants*

Other toxins produced by different molds are of equal concern for children's health. These include toxins that occur in food as a result of mold growth. Some of this can occur during the storage of grains such as wheat, corn, oats and barley. Most of the exposure occurs by eating food with the contaminants. These toxins include aflatoxin, ochratoxin, T-2 toxin and fusarium toxin. While aflatoxin has long been known as a contaminant of peanut butter, the public may be less familiar with others that are fungal toxins. They can be quite potent and for this reason even small amounts can be harmful. Their action is not restricted solely to the immune system. For example, aflatoxin B-1 toxin is known to cause liver cancer. Many mycotoxins are known to depress both cell-mediated immunity and antibody responses. However, some mycotoxins may also contribute to allergic and autoimmune diseases.

Exposure to aflatoxin during embryonic development was reported to suppress cell-mediated immunity in the offspring. With another mycotoxin, T-2, gestational exposure in animals produced atrophy of the thymus, altered lymphocyte populations and seemed to target the stem cells (progenitor cells) of the immune system. The results suggest that mycotoxins are a serious hazard for the young with suppressed cell-mediated immune functions (anticancer and antiviral responses) as a likely outcome.

23. *Timing of Childhood Vaccination*

Vaccinations are an effective way to prevent many life-threatening childhood diseases. They are effective in protecting children from specific diseases (e.g., diphtheria, pertussis, tetanus, measles, mumps, rubella) that the vaccines were designed to address. In fact, they are likely to be among the most effective therapeutics against illness that a child will ever receive. However, the timing of childhood vaccinations and even the combinations of vaccine components included in vaccines are not necessarily determined on the basis of the optimum immune health of the child. Instead, they may reflect other priorities. Recent studies suggest that the timing of some childhood vaccinations may be a contributing factor to the recent rise in allergies and childhood asthma. In some countries vaccines are now administered shortly after birth while the immune system is undergoing critical maturation. It now appears that the goal of giving the child the earliest possible chance to see a vaccine may create a considerable side effect; higher risk of allergies and childhood asthma. This may be a result of the immaturity of the innate immune system at birth coupled with the fact that the newborn is emerging from the Th2-biased environment of the pregnancy.

Parents should discuss this issue of timing of vaccinations with their pediatrician in reaching a decision at what age their children will be vaccinated to optimize overall immune health.

24. *Caesarian Section (Mode of Birth Delivery)*

Several studies within the past five years have reported that the mode of birth delivery influences both neonatal immune status and health risks. Children delivered by Cesarean section (C-section) have an increased risk for developing asthma and allergies when compared to those babies delivered vaginally. Immune parameters also reflect this differential risk. Babies delivered by C-section have reduced levels of the cytokine interferon-gamma (a Th1 cytokine) and elevated levels of IL-4 (a Th2 cytokine) when compared with vaginally-delivered babies. This suggests that the C-section babies are stuck in a more Th2 skewed mode of immune function (allergy-promoting) with the needed maturation of Th1 immune capacity (antiviral, anticancer) lagging behind.

The reason that birth delivery mode affects risk of asthma and allergies is not yet established. However, several possibilities exist. First, the physical process and challenge of vaginal delivery may provide the baby's immune system with certain chemical signals that aid further maturation of the baby's immune system. A second possibility is that a certain level of microbial exposure occurs as the baby is born vaginally that is absent with a C-section delivery. Since it is known that exposure to bacteria cell wall components helps immune maturation, this brief environmental exposure in the birth canal may stimulate the newborn's immune system to mature. Finally, preoperative prophylactic administration of antibiotics to the mother is used in some C-section procedures. Since exposure of the child to antibiotics before and just after birth is known to promote asthma, this could be an indirect way in which C-section delivery affects the risk of childhood asthma.

Regardless of the mechanism for affecting health risk, parents will want to discuss birth delivery mode options with their physicians. There are significant medical reasons why C-sections would be recommended. But it is important that parents understand the potential health implications for their children. All immediate and long-term risks should be discussed with their medical specialists.

25. *Ultraviolet Radiation*

Excessive ultraviolet radiation can be immunosuppressive both in the skin and systemically. This seems to be mediated via vitamin D receptors on immune cells. However, a certain level of vitamin D is needed for good immune function, which is difficult to maintain since the human body does not produce vitamin D in the absence of adequate sun exposure. Plus, low vitamin D levels are associated with allergic and autoimmune disease in children and certain cancers in adults. This is a clear example where vitamin D is needed both prenatally and in childhood. But sunburn (over exposure to ultraviolet light) can contribute to a higher risk of immunosuppression as well as skin cancer in later life. Obviously, a balance in sun exposure without sun block is needed, one in which enough sun exposure is possible but not so long that a burn is initiated. As a substitute, fish liver oils are usually high in vitamin D. The thing to watch with fish liver oils is to be sure that the fish liver oil is derived from mercury-free sources.

Conclusions

This chapter has discussed the Top 25 environmental risk factors that contribute to DIT and an increased risk of immune-based diseases. Not every factor is equal in risk. For a few, there remains some uncertainty. But we have attempted to provide some prioritization among this Top 25 group.

Obviously, the ease of protecting pregnant moms and young children from these environmental exposures and conditions will vary from factor to factor. Some are easier than others. For example, it is going to be easier for a parent to know if the pregnant mom has been prescribed antibiotics than knowing with certainty that a newly purchased toy is free of lead. In the case of new drugs, the specialized risk for the pregnant woman or young child may not be obvious. In these cases, it never hurts to ask what immunological safety information exists.

We hope that this list of high priority risk factors will better prepare expecting and new parents with information useful for creating an immune-supportive environment for their children.

Overview of the Top 25 Risks

- Our Top 25 Risks and your own exposure worries may not be identical. That's not a problem. The information here and in Chapter 17 and the Appendix is only a reference guide for your use.
- Every risk factor you protect against tilts the odds in favor of your child's immune system.
- Your child is unique and these risks are based on populations of children.

Chapter 17 — Other Risk Factors

Introduction

The previous chapter presented information on the Top 25 Risks for the developing immune system. In this chapter, we include numerous other chemical, drug and microbial risk factors for the developing immune system that deserve the attention of parents and physicians. Not all factors will be of equal concern for each child. For example, some represent more significant occupational and neighborhood-dependent exposures. A given factor may have significance for one family but not necessarily another. However, having this checklist of additional hazards available should arm parents with the information they need to better protect their child's immune system.

The risk factors are listed below in alphabetical order. Details of these are found in the Appendix.

Aluminum Compounds — The most common metal found in the earth's crust.

Asbestos — A fibrous mineral material that was once used for insulation and as a fire retardant.

Benzene — Benzene is an organic chemical in the category called aromatic hydrocarbons.

Beryllium — A relatively strong and light metal that occurs naturally as an element.

1-Bromopropane (1-BP) — Dry Cleaning Agent — 1-BP (also called n-propyl-bromide) has become a popular solvent for cleaning.

Chlordane — Chlordane is a member of the family of organochlorine pesticides.

DEET (N,N,-diethyl-*m*-toluamide) — An active agent in some insect repellants.

Diazinon — An organophosphate insecticide once used extensively by gardeners.

Diazepam — Diazepam (first marketed under the trade name, Valium) is a drug that has been used to treat anxiety, seizures, muscle spasms, sleep problems, and drug withdrawal symptoms.

Ethylene Glycol — An alcohol-like substance that is used in antifreeze for cars.

Gold — Gold salts have been used in some medications.

Lindane (Lice Treatment) — Lindane is used in medications for the treatment of lice and scabies parasite infestations.

Mancozeb — A carbamate derivative compound that is used extensively as a fungicide.

New Carpets — This is an often overlooked source of chemical exposure.

Organotins — Organotins include several different tin-based compounds that are found in anti-fouling marine paints and are used in the production of polyvinyl chloride (PVC) tubes and bottles.

Other Organophosphate Pesticides — Other organophosphate pesticides (OP) include parathion, chlorpyrifos, malathion.

Palladium — Palladium is from the same group of metals as platinum.

Phosphamidon — Phosphamidon is another organophosphate insecticide

Platinum — Platinum is used in jewelry as well as in catalytic converters in automobiles.

Polybrominated Biphenyls (Flame Retardants) — PBBs are flame retardant chemicals.

Pthalates — A group of chemicals added to plastics to make them more flexible.

Propanil — Propanil is one of the more commonly used herbicides in the United States.

Pyrethroid Insecticides — Used to control a variety of insects particularly mosquitoes.

Respiratory Syncytial Virus (RSV) Infection — A common virus that infects the airways.

Silica Dust — Silica is a naturally occurring substance that is found in rocks and sand.

Tattoos — Tattoos may contain a variety of toxins that can present potential problems for immune cells.

Therapeutic Proteins — Therapeutic proteins are proteins that are engineered in the lab for pharmaceutical use.

Vinyl Chloride — Vinyl chloride is used in the production of polyvinyl chloride (PVC) which is included in a variety of plastic products including bottles.

Conclusions

A wide range of immune risk factors are presented in both the prior Top 25 Risks chapter, the current chapter and the Appendix. It should be noted that exposures may occur from every route (e.g., air, food, and skin contact). Health risks vary from increased susceptibility to infectious disease, to a heightened risk of allergies, inflammation, tissue damage and autoimmune disease. For the most part, the diseases are both serious and persistent. They can arise shortly after exposure or lie dormant then spring to life in adulthood.

In the next chapter we will discuss how some factors appear to act as triggers of disease for an immune system that is already developmentally damaged.

Chapter 18 — Postnatal Triggers of Disease — Infections

Introduction

Many different environmental risk factors contribute to childhood immune dysfunction and immune-related disease in children. But the precise nature of these contributions can differ among the risk factors (toxic chemicals and drugs, diet, psychological or physical stress and infectious agents). We have already discussed how some toxic chemicals and drugs can damage the developing immune system during prenatal and neonatal life making it dysfunctional throughout a child's life. By "causing" immune dysfunction via immune insults, these factors produce the equivalent of an immunological land mine. The land mine is hidden and quietly waiting to be revealed. Often, it and its danger only become apparent once it has been triggered. Toxicants like alcohol, cigarette smoke, dioxin, PCBs, some pesticides, heavy metals and endocrine disrupting compounds damage the developing immune system and "cause" this childhood land mine to form. But exactly when and where the immunological land mine will explode can depend upon other risk factors: the triggers.

How Triggers Work

These other immune risk factors play a different role in producing immune-related disease in children. These are the "triggers" or final steps in producing immune-related diseases. They will set off our immune dysfunctional land mine. They effectively step on the immune land mine and trigger an explosion of serious disease. You may be asking, how can they do this? In most cases, they do this by simply challenging the damaged immune system. The existing damage means that the immune system can't respond normally, and the abnormal immune response produces the disease. The land mine of hidden damage was already there. But the disease will not show up until the land mine is triggered. "Triggers" are usually the final step in the sequence of steps by which developmental immunotoxicity shows up as serious disease in children.

Several different risk factors can serve as triggers. But infectious agents (viruses, bacteria, fungi, parasites) are the most important category of triggers of immune-dysfunction-based disease. They simply challenge the child's immune system and when that system has been previously damaged, unanticipated diseases can result. The genetic background of the child is important too and because of this, not every child is at equal risk to the causes and triggers of diseases associated with developmental immunotoxicity.

Diseases That Can Have Infections as Triggers

Virtually every category of immune-based disease has either a well-established or a suspected infection that can trigger the disease in those susceptible individuals (individuals with environmentally-caused immune dysfunction and/or genetic predisposition). The disease categories with triggers include: allergic diseases, autoimmune diseases, inflammatory diseases, life-threatening infections (e.g., bacterial pneumonia) and cancer. Whether a given disease is likely to develop is dependent upon: 1) the nature of the underlying immune dysfunction in the child and 2) exposure to the proper trigger (specific virus, bacteria, etc.) for the disease. If the child is able to avoid the trigger, then the disease may be delayed or prevented from ever developing. However, this action alone would not defuse or remove the underlying immune dysfunction (the land mine) in the child.

Examples of some immune-based diseases and their proposed triggers are shown in Table 18.1.

Table 18.1. Immune-based diseases and their proposed triggers.

Disease or Condition	Proposed Triggering Infection(s)
Asthma	Respiratory syncytial virus, rhinovirus
Bacterial pneumonia	Influenza virus
Childhood leukemia (e.g., acute lymphoblastic leukemia)	Unidentified common infections
Juvenile arthritis (in girls)	Unidentified infections in the first year of life
Multiple sclerosis	Viruses (possibly the Epstein Barr virus).
Repeated ear infections and complications	Streptococcus bacteria (and other bacteria)
Type 1 diabetes	Enteroviruses

Information from: Dietert R. Distinguishing environmental causes of immune dysfunction from pediatric triggers of disease. *Open Pediatr Med J* 3: 38–44, 2009.

The take-home lesson from Table 18.1 is that many important immune-based diseases can be triggered in children and young adults by relatively common infections. It may not be possible or even practical to completely avoid these infections throughout a lifetime. Therefore, a more effective way to reduce the risk of these diseases is to: 1) avoid developmental immune toxicity and the immune damage that establishes the land mine or 2) correct the immune damage in the child before the child encounters a trigger. At present, avoiding the damage appears to be easier, more cost effective and more certain than correction of underlying pediatric immune dysfunction.

Overview of Postnatal Infections as Triggers

- Childhood infections are probably the most important triggers of immune dysfunction-based diseases.
- Most infections are not the primary cause of immune dysfunction-related diseases.
- Instead, they reveal the existence of underlying immune dysfunction in childhood and trigger the onset of diseases.

Chapter 19 — Postnatal Triggers of Disease — Vaccinations

Introduction

Childhood Vaccinations and Health Risks

Here is the topic everyone has been waiting for. It is controversial and is likely to continue to be controversial for a while. In fact, it may be one reason why you bought this book. It is a topic we have engaged in a prior peer-reviewed science article concerning the developing immune system and disease and have discussed in technical jargon in a book on immunotoxicity testing for safety of the childhood immune system. In this chapter we will try to shed some light on the issue and arm you with a few useful questions to ask as you and your pediatrician design a strategy for your child's overall health. In the end we will also give you the "What would you do?" answer from the authors.

Commonly-Encountered Vaccines

It can be easy to forget the real toll that childhood infectious diseases took as recently as the 1950s. The success of vaccines in dramatically reducing many of the common childhood and adult infectious diseases is stunning. Among the vaccines that are used today are: hemophilus influenzae type B (Hib), diphtheria, varicella (pertussis), human papilloma virus (HPV), hepatitis A and B, poliovirus, measles, mumps, rubella, pneumococcal vaccine, meningococcal vaccine, zoster, rotavirus, rabies and yellow fever. Note that the CDC recommends against several of these for pregnant or breastfeeding women. In the following sections we will discuss both the benefits and the immunological risks of vaccines.

The Benefits

Vaccinations have been one of the modern medical breakthroughs that have saved and continue to save countless lives. The vast majority of vaccines are extremely effective although depending upon disease, the effectiveness does vary. Much of this book advocates the benefits of prevention, and that is precisely what vaccines are designed to do, prevent disease. By the early 1950s, new polio cases in the U.S. alone had risen to between 20,000–55,000 per year. Considering the fact that the disease can produce extensive, lasting paralysis and sometimes death, this was a devastating childhood-onset illness that was expanding in our population. The impact of polio on children that survived ranged from significantly impaired mobility to whole body paralysis that required a lifetime of living inside an iron lung just to breathe. The development and use of polio vaccines have effectively eradicated this disease in much of the world. Only where vaccination is incomplete in children does the disease continue to exist. The results for the other vaccine types have been equally successful, and thousands of children no longer die or live with crippling disabilities as a result of these serious diseases.

Vaccines usually come in several varieties: 1) killed virus, 2) live, but altered (called attenuated) virus that does not produce the disease, 3) DNA or subunit vaccines that are designed to help our immune system see only part of the virus, but with the virus protein synthesized inside our own cells or 4) pieces of a bacterium or its toxin. An example from this last category of vaccines is the tetanus vaccine that is given to protect against the toxin produced by the bacteria that causes tetanus. As previously mentioned in Chapter 4, significant exposure to this toxin produces a paralysis involving muscles and nerves commonly known as lockjaw. Death can result from problems with breathing or with the heart. The vaccine has a history that dates back to the 1920s. The botulism bacterium that produces tetanus toxin is present in nature, and a very small infection can produce enough toxin to create suffocating paralysis. In this case, the vaccine used is made of inactivated toxin. The antibodies we produce as a result of vaccination bind up any toxin we might encounter so that it cannot reach our tissues. However, we do need a booster about every ten years. In the past few decades, the tetanus vaccine has been mixed with diphtheria and pertussis vaccine when given to children. The mixture is commonly known as DPT vaccine.

Talk to the Animals

If human vaccines have a long track record of examining their benefits and risks, so do vaccines developed for our pets and food-producing animals. In fact, it is likely that chicken would not be the word's preeminent animal protein source but for numerous highly effective vaccines against diseases such as Newcastle's disease, infectious bronchitis, infectious bursal disease and Marek's disease. Why is this so? For example, virtually every chicken in the world is exposed to the Marek's disease virus, a herpes virus. The disease itself is devastating and produces both cancer and nerve damage. Marek's disease vaccines developed at places like Cornell University are critical for chickens to survive until they are mature enough to reproduce. It is safe to say that this vaccine has been for chickens what the polio vaccine has been for humans.

Similarly, most pet owners are well aware of the effectiveness of rabies, parvovirus and distemper vaccines in dogs and feline distemper and leukemia virus vaccines in cats. Our pets' health depends upon the development and use of these vaccines. Many animal vaccines work exceptionally well and keep our pets healthy and our food affordable. But to borrow a phrase from a famous Cornelian, Dr. Carl Sagan, with "billions and billions" of, in this case, vaccinated chickens, dogs, cats and other animals, we have also learned about the nature of potential side effects and risks that can be associated with widespread vaccine use. This is why it is important to ask the right questions about vaccines and to understand both the benefits and the risks.

Ask the Right Questions

Obviously, vaccines do a world of good. But are they risk-free? No. The risk is above zero as it is for most things, but it is small for most vaccines.

Can allergic reactions and other adverse side effects occur in at least some children? Yes. Will they occur in your child? We don't know for certain. Do we know all the risks involved with vaccinations? Probably not. Are there side effects we usually don't test for, but should? Absolutely.

The Risks of Vaccinations

Timing of vaccinations and immune status

For example, yellow fever vaccine is not recommended for infants six months of age and under because of the risk of developing viral encephalomyelitis (brain inflammation). Additionally, pregnant women should not be vaccinated because of the risk of infection to the fetus. These two age-based prohibitions for certain vaccinations reflect the importance of immune maturation in the likely reactions to a vaccine. Whether an immune system is fully matured or is inappropriately skewed in function can influence both the effectiveness of the immune response to vaccines and the potential for unhealthy side effects that can occur with some vaccinations. A discussion of the timing of infant vaccinations and risk of asthma was previously covered in the chapters on postnatal strategies and the Top 25 Risks. Parents should discuss the timing of childhood vaccinations with their pediatrician.

Unintended immunomodulation

We know that certain infections can predispose children for a second illness. For example, early and severe infection with respiratory syncytial virus (RSV) or rhinovirus can increase the risk of the child developing asthma (discussed in Chapter 18). Similarly, an infection with influenza can increase the chances of bacterial pneumonia so that it requires treatment with antibiotics. Would it then be surprising if some live viral vaccines that are designed to produce a mild protective infection might cause unintended immunomodulation as well? Not at all. In fact, the animal vaccine literature is full of examples that are very similar. For example, in a 1992 study in Israel that used several different Marek's disease vaccines that had all been proven to protect against the disease, researchers found that some commercial vaccines significantly increased the risk of bacterial infection in young chicks while others provided viral protection without the side effect of increased bacterial disease risk. Because this difference in vaccine response occurred in chickens with the same background, eating the same food and living in the same housing, the side effect of susceptibility to bacterial infection was due to the vaccine. So the potential is there for some vaccines to modulate the immune system in unanticipated ways. All the vaccines were good for protecting against Marek's disease. But some were not good for the chick's overall immune system.

The key to better vaccine safety is not just looking at whether the vaccine works against the target disease but also looking at whether it changes the immune system in such a way that it increases other health risks. Prior to that study, no one had a clue that some Marek's vaccinations might cause the chicks to have problems fighting off bacteria.

In another example, adult horses are frequently vaccinated against a herpes virus disease using a killed form of the virus (to avoid fetal risk when the live virus is used). Frequently, the vaccine is given two to three times per year; but for some horse facilities it is given more often. In this case, giving more shots per year seems to have unanticipated health risks. Researchers observed that horses that were given boosters four times a year (instead of two to three per year) were more likely to develop neurological problems if they encountered the actual virus. In that case, more vaccinations are not better. Instead, it can lead to a greater chance of serious health problems. The exact mechanism for this side-effect is not known. But it emphasizes the importance of understanding precisely what a vaccination does to the entire immune system and overall immune function and not just whether you see antibodies produced to the target virus or bacterium.

Could similar unintended immune changes happen in some children? It is certainly possible. Just as infections appear to be a trigger of asthma and autoimmune disease (discussed in Chapter 18), some vaccinations have the potential to push the immune system of certain children into a place where other diseases might become an issue. If you don't believe this then ask yourself why the Hemophilus influenzae B (Hib) vaccination has been found to protect children from childhood leukemia? The vaccine seems to push the immune system to a place where the pre-leukemic lymphocytes do not progress to leukemia. In this case it is a good thing.

But nobody knew that the vaccine was making those changes to immune cells. Of course, the reverse scenario is just as possible where some vaccinations could increase the risk of undesirable or ineffective immune responses in some children.

Why is this a potential trigger?

You may be asking why childhood vaccinations are being considered more as a possible trigger for disease in some children rather than a prominent "cause." Part of the reason is that many of the possible adverse effects from vaccines seem to be dependent upon genetic predisposition and past environmental toxin exposures. Much like the infections discussed in Chapter 18, vaccinations are more likely to be the last step in a DIT process leading to disease rather than the stand-alone cause of chronic immune-based disease.

Vaccines or Additives

There has been considerable concern about vaccine carriers and preservatives, among them the mercury-containing compound, thimerasol. Mercury is a very serious neurological and immunological toxin. But many of the adverse effects thought to be linked to thimerasol (e.g., autism) are diagnosed early in the infant (e.g., by 18 months of age). This means that any environmental effect can occur anytime prior to 18 months of age. If early vaccinations are involved in early-life onset conditions like autism, they are more likely to act as triggers, similar to how infections trigger autoimmune disease. It seems less likely to be a stand-alone cause. That is not to say that triggers are ok or that exposure to mercury at any time is a good idea. You do not want your child exposed to harmful levels of mercury; not in vaccines, dental amalgams nor light bulbs.

It is useful to recognize that diseases even in childhood may involve multiple earlier critical windows of vulnerability. Early immune disruption can play out as later disease and many of those diseases take time to emerge. A stunning example is atherosclerosis, a disease generally associated with middle and old age. But atherosclerosis, a disease of aging, has its origins in early life. In fact, biomarkers for atherosclerosis can be detected in children, but it takes years for the disease to actually develop. Many cancers, such as breast cancer, are affected by childhood events, but the concerns themselves can take decades to emerge and are often considered "adult" diseases.

With autism and autism spectrum disorders (ASD), much of the focus has been on the postnatal environment and any "events" just prior to diagnosis of the condition in children. But it seems likely that the most sensitive period for neurological insult occurs prenatally. This is supported by many of the best models of autism and ASD, which combine prenatal environmental insult with genetic predisposition to affect neurological development.

Allergic Reactions

A final unintended outcome of vaccination can be an allergic reaction to some component of the vaccine preparation. Ironically, this is a side effect that is well-acknowledged by vaccine companies, physicians and patients (unlike unintended immunomodulation). Fortunately, the side effect is relatively rare so the risk is relatively low. But parents do need to be aware that allergic reactions to vaccines can happen just as they can occur in the case of drug allergies.

"What Would We Do?"

We promised this section at the beginning of the chapter. Now that we have outlined for you both the positives of vaccinations and the problems, it's time for us to present what we would do. If it helps, we're both parents of grown children. So this topic is pertinent for us as well.

The normal North American vaccination schedule is two, four and six months of age for DPT. In Japan the vaccination schedule is usually six to nine months with no DPT before three months of age. At an earlier point in time, Japan didn't vaccinate for DPT before two years old, and this late age was associated with both an increased rate of pertussis but with a lower rate of asthma. This tells us that timing is important. Not too soon and not too late. Finding a happy median of when to give DPT is important in protecting the child from both pertussis and from a lifetime of allergies and asthma.

To begin with, as soon as we knew we were expecting a baby, we would seek out a pediatrician, perhaps one that was more open to integrative medicine, at least more open to working in partnership with parents on their child's immune health. We would set up an appointment for a consultation with this pediatrician, and we would come armed with family history, questions and a few pieces of literature. We would open a discussion about vaccinations right up front. It's too important to be left until a later date when as new parents we're sleep-deprived from being up with our new bundle of joy.

Our conversation with the pediatrician might go something like this. "We believe that vaccinations are important. We're aware of the suffering children and their parents went through before vaccines were common and how many children either died or were disabled for life by diseases. We want our child's health protected. However, we are very concerned about what's in some vaccines, such as thimerasol, how many diseases are being vaccinated against at one time, and how early vaccines are given. We've been searching the literature and have some articles that support our concerns that we'd appreciate your reading. If we could work together to create a vaccination schedule for our child that optimizes our child's immune health, we would appreciate it."

Then, we would give the doctor a couple of articles and, most likely this book now that this resource is also available. One such article might be "Delay in diphtheria, pertussis, tetanus vaccination is associated with a reduced risk of childhood asthma," by McDonald KL *et al.* in the *Journal of Allergy and Clinical Immunology* 2008 Mar;121(3):626–631. This article and several others have opened a lot of discussion on the subject of vaccination schedule. While the scientists search for confirmation of the findings, the fact is that the study has created reasonable doubt, and it's that reasonable doubt that makes it important to consider all options when looking at the timing of when vaccinations are given.

Putting Causes and Triggers Together

Because infections, vaccinations and other stressors can all be triggers of immune-based disease in certain children, it is useful to visualize how

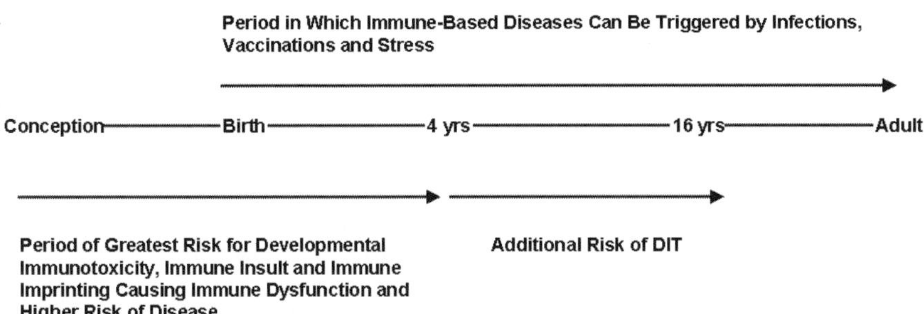

Figure 19.1. Developmental immunotoxicity and triggers of immune-based disease.

this fits in with DIT (causes of immune dysfunction). This is shown in Figure 19.1. Once the immune dysfunctional state is established, a variety of triggers can lead to disease.

Conclusions

Vaccines have been a modern-day miracle in protecting our children against deadly diseases. They continue to protect countless of the world's population against preventable illness, and our children should be protected against preventable life-threatening diseases.

However, vaccines are not without some risk. The most likely risk appears to be a result of unexpected or unintended immune responses. The genetic background of individuals may influence such responses. However, prior environmentally-induced immune dysfunction and lack of complete maturity of the immune system are two additional concerns. Part of the solution is clear. We should fully understand the safety of vaccines. This means understanding not just if they will produce needed immune responses against the virus or bacterium but also if certain vaccines can undesirably change other immune response capabilities of our children. Additionally, we should have science-based information as to the optimum timing of vaccinations for our children's overall health. Parents and pediatricians play an important role in this solution as their opinions count. They are the customers in the service industry of childhood vaccinations.

Overview of Postnatal Vaccines as Triggers

- Vaccines are effective in preventing many serious childhood and adult diseases.
- Children should be protected against preventable diseases.
- Some vaccines may have the potential to cause immunomodulatation in some individuals.
- Legitimate safety questions exist about the timing of some childhood vaccinations.
- Vaccine use should optimize total immune health and safety testing should ensure this is the case for our children.

Chapter 20 — Dietary Factors that Affect the Immune System

Introduction

Diet, is among the defining factors that help to set your baby's immune system on its life course. For that reason, careful attention to maternal diet during pregnancy and the diet of your infant or adolescent child is an essential part of effectively managing your child's immune system.

There are many dietary factors that directly affect the immune system. Some of them like sugar are more negative given the amounts normally consumed, while others like specific vitamins tend to provide a boost. Some of these substances like vitamins C and D, the human body cannot manufacture and needs to derive them from external sources. We will take a look at a range of dietary factors that research says affect the immune system in general with a focus on the developing immune system.

Vitamins

Vitamins in general have been getting a lot of attention over the past few years because research has increased our understanding of the essential roles many of them have in modulating a number of immune processes.

A —

Vitamin A has long been known to influence the immune system. Scientists found that it has an impact on lymphocyte activation and proliferation, aids in T helper cell differentiation, helps with tissue-specific lymphocyte homing, helps with the production of specific antibody isotypes and aids in regulating immune responses. Researchers now think it is useful to prevent and/or treat inflammation and autoimmunity. People who are deficient in vitamin A have greater difficulty fighting off infections and complications of infectious diseases. Even a mild degree of vitamin A deficiency may increase a child's risk of developing respiratory infections and diarrhea. Vitamin A deficiency also decreases survival odds during a severe illness.

Since this is a vitamin that is stored in the liver, care must be taken to ingest enough without getting too much, an area where "the dose makes the poison." And in some Western societies with high dietary fat intake, we can easily get too much of these fat-soluble vitamins in our diet.

Betacarotene —

Betacarotene is one of the carotenoids, highly pigmented (red, orange, yellow) compounds naturally present in many fruits, grains, vegetable oils, and vegetables. All forms of betacarotene are considered to be important as provitamins that are converted into active vitamin A. The carotenoids possess antioxidant properties and are also involved in the synthesis of certain glycoproteins. They are particularly good for dealing with viral infections, both acute and chronic. As with vitamin A, it is quite possible to ingest too much betacarotene for your immune system.

B5 or Pantothentic acid —

Pantothentic acid is a B vitamin that plays an important role in immune system function. It can powerfully protect against infections and help the body withstand stressful conditions. Pantothentic acid stimulates the adrenal cortex and participates in the production of energy. It also helps maintain a healthy digestive tract as well as protects against the harmful effects of antibiotics. It may also help reduce inflammation stemming from disorders like allergies, asthma, lupus and psoriasis. Pantothentic acid occurs in all sources of food (plants and animals).

C —

Vitamin C is probably the most well-known vitamin. According to a study presented at the 60th Anniversary Meeting of the American Academy of Allergy, Asthma and Immunology, daily doses of vitamin C can boost the immune system and help protect against viral infections. Large doses can even decrease the incidence and severity of the common cold. vitamin C intake increases the numbers of natural killer cells present in the blood as well as their ability to make antiviral compounds. The number of T cells appears to remain the same, but those present are more activated following higher vitamin C ingestion. They also produce significantly more interferon-gamma (a Th1 virus-fighting cytokine) and less IL-4 (a Th2 cytokine). In this study, higher immune antiviral activity was achieved in the study after only two weeks of participants taking 1g/day Vitamin C supplement. On top of its antiviral activities, vitamin C is known as one of the top antioxidants.

One to two gram doses of vitamin C per day have been shown to reduce asthma symptoms significantly. Sufficient amounts of vitamin C in the blood can protect the joints of rheumatoid arthritis patients from further damage. It may also strengthen artery walls in a way that prevents atherosclerosis largely by preventing white blood cells from adhering to them.

What is nice about vitamin C is that, because it is water soluble, it's more difficult to get too much compared with other vitamins. Usually, what isn't needed is simply flushed from the system or excreted.

D —

According to the Archives of Internal Medicine, the majority of Americans are vitamin D deficient. This, in turn, negatively impacts immune function and cardiovascular health while increasing cancer risk. In fact, vitamin D deficiency is associated with inflammation because too little allows levels of tumor necrosis factor-alpha (TNF-alpha) to increase.

Elevated levels of TNF-alpha play a role in initiating heart disease, multiple sclerosis and rheumatoid arthritis. Healthy levels of vitamin D help keep inflammation in check and aid the immune system in mounting an adequate response to a challenge.

Vitamin D is unusual in the world of vitamins because it is actually a hormone, though not one that we can synthesize ourselves. We need either sunshine on non-sunscreened skin (for at least 20–30 minutes per day, but not long enough to produce a burn). Otherwise, we must get our vitamin D from foods. At this time the old 1997 values for daily requirements are being revised to reflect recent research particularly that performed by Harvard School of Public Health researchers. Their study says that adequate daily intake for adults should begin at 1,000 IU per day.

Most immune cells have the receptor for vitamin D, including T cells and antigen-presenting cells like dendritic cells and macrophages. Adequate levels of vitamin D appear to enhance innate immunity and may prevent the development of autoimmunity.

There is now direct evidence that vitamin D prevents inflammation, both that found naturally in wounds and that as a result of chemical intervention. Researchers are now looking at the possibility of using vitamin D to control autoimmune diseases that are thought to be caused by overactive cytokine responses, such as autoimmune diabetes, multiple sclerosis and inflammatory bowel disease.

There has been some concern that taking daily supplements of vitamin D could cause toxicity. However, research has shown that toxicity isn't seen until doses reach 40,000 IU taken daily for an extended period of time. That figure is just for ingested supplements. When it comes to the amount of vitamin D derived from sun exposure, a toxic level has yet to be determined, but the risk from sunburn is the foremost concern.

Too little vitamin D during pregnancy is a significant risk factor for the infant. Vitamin D deficiencies both impair the developing immune system and skew the immune responses toward promoting allergies.

E —

Researchers have found that vitamin E, an antioxidant, may help maintain the immune system as we age. When participants in a clinical trial took as little as 200 mg a day for four months, they had stronger responses to vaccines for hepatitis B and tetanus than did those taking a placebo. In other words, their immune systems responded better when challenged. Worth noting was the fact that 200 mg seemed to be the optimum dose because those who took a lower dose, 60 mg, and those who took the higher dose, 800 mg, didn't do as well. Again, as with the other dietary factors, there is a dose range that is optimal for the immune system.

Some of the ways in which vitamin E may impact the immune system is by enhancing the behavior of naïve T cells (T cells that haven't been exposed to an antigen). They reproduce better and produce more IL-2 (a T cell growth factor cytokine). This action bolsters the immune system and makes it more effective when responding to challenge.

Tocotrienols, which are members of the vitamin E family, have been found to have very attractive anticancer properties. Gamma- and delta-tocotrienols appear to accumulate in cancer cells and promote the death of tumors.

Minerals

Humans and other living organisms require four major elements: carbon, hydrogen, nitrogen and oxygen. Dietary minerals are basically the other elements required for life. They support many interactions in the body including: 1) enzyme action to eliminate toxins and 2) support for hemoglobin to carry oxygen. Often these are placed under the category of micronutrients, although micronutrients also include vitamins and fats. Many minerals are essential and are required for life.

Iodine —

Iodine is a naturally occurring trace element most known for its affects on the thyroid. However, it is also necessary for a healthy immune system and has been used therapeutically as an antibacterial, antiparasitic, antiviral and anticancer substance. In research, iodine, in doses above the recommended daily allowance (RDA), promoted cell death in tumor cells. While table salt is generally enriched with iodine, it may be a form that is less available to your child's body. Instead, the ocean is a more abundant source for iodine, which is found in seaweed and fish (though many ocean fish also have high levels of mercury). Animal feeds are also often iodized.

Like tocotrienols, iodine appears to accumulate in diseased tissues where it becomes a part of a potent antimicrobial process that quickly kills bacteria, viruses, fungi and other micro-organisms. Iodine in combination with peroxidase and hydrogen peroxide has potent antimicrobial activities against bacteria, fungi (including several species of candida), viruses and mycoplasma and is highly toxic to HIV-1.

Selenium —

Selenium was used as an example in an earlier chapter of this book. It is an important antioxidant that is usually found in the soil in different regions around the world. Some of its antioxidant actions are mediated through glutathione peroxidases. Its primary antioxidant effect seems to be in the extracellular space (outside the cells), specifically in the G.I. tract. Selenium appears to influence both innate and acquired immunity. Lymphocytes that are deficient in selenium are less able to proliferate in response to a challenge, and macrophages are also impacted when selenium levels are too low. IgM, IgG and IgA levels are decreased when there is not enough selenium in the system. The lack of selenium in the systems of asthmatics causes neutrophils to adhere in greater numbers, which can cause greater inflammatory damage to the lining of the lungs. Selenium toxicity was discussed in prior chapters.

Zinc —

Zinc is an essential mineral that is important for cell metabolism. The body needs a daily supply because it has no zinc storage system. It is particularly important for normal growth and development during pregnancy, childhood and adolescence. Zinc is essential for appropriate immune function. Even mild to moderate levels of zinc deficiency can weaken macrophage and neutrophil functions and natural killer cell activity. Low zinc levels reduce lymphocyte proliferation responses to mitogens, which may explain why low zinc status is associated with greater susceptibility to pneumonia and other infections. In the common cold, researchers hypothesize that zinc may directly inhibit the rhinovirus from binding and replicating in nasal mucosa. Plus, they believe it may reduce inflammation. Zinc serves as a portion of many different enzymes needed for proper immune function. There is more known about the role of zinc in adults and the elderly than in the young. However, zinc deficiency can occur and will result in immunosuppression along with increased susceptibility to infections. So ensuring adequate zinc intake either through diet or with zinc supplements is important for your child's immune system.

Unlike the situation with vitamin C, it is easier to get too much zinc. Zinc toxicity usually begins with doses greater than 150–450 mg per day.

Amino Acids

Amino acids are the building blocks of life. Without them, no proteins or cells in the body would be created. Specific amino acids are the basis for DNA. Some are more specialized than others, and particular ones seem to have more impact on the immune system than others.

Arginine —

Arginine is one of the amino acids that is important for a healthy immune system. Dietary arginine can increase the weight of the thymus, something that researchers have directly correlated to an increase in the number of thymic T lymphocytes. It can also increase the number of T cells that are released by the thymus. Arginine can increase the proliferation of peripheral monocytes and lymphocytes and improve cell-mediated immune reactions. This amino acid also plays a role in the creation of nitric oxide, which is important in inflammation and immunity. Nitric oxide is produced by macrophages and neutrophils and can kill bacteria and tumor cells and affect the activity of other immune cells.

Glutamine —

Glutamine is known as a "conditionally essential amino acid." That means that, while it is normally found in the body, when someone is under stress, be it illness or psychological stress, or has surgery, the body gets depleted of glutamine. In conjunction with N-acetyl cysteine (NAC), glutamine forms the most important compound in the body, glutathione (a previously mentioned antioxidant). Glutamine is used to make the proteins that are the building blocks of the body and is used to carry excess ammonia out of the body. It nourishes the cells of the intestinal lining and the stomach and is the primary fuel source for lymphocytes, macrophages and neutrophils. Research has shown that lymphocytes depend on glutamine in order to synthesize IL-2 and macrophages depend on it to synthesize IL-1. The ability of macrophages to phagocytose (ingest and metabolize antigens) intruders is highly influenced by the amount of glutamine available. Depletion of glutamine regularly leads to immunosuppression, an observation that has been seen in cases of trauma (e.g., sepsis, injury, burns and surgery) as well as in athletes who over-train.

Histidine —

Histidine is an amino acid that is found in hemoglobin in abundance. It is needed for the production of both red and white blood cells. Histamine, which helps regulate the physiological function of the gut as well as acts as a neurotransmitter that is important for sleep, is derived directly from histidine. This amino acid has been used to treat rheumatoid arthritis, allergies, ulcers and anemia.

Lysine —

Lysine is an essential amino acid, meaning that it cannot be made by the body, yet the body depends on it for good health. It plays an essential role in the production of carnitine, which is necessary for energy production, and helps the body absorb and conserve calcium. Lysine also helps the body form collagen, which is part of the connective tissues in the body. Researchers have tested lysine for the possibility of pain control by pairing it with painkillers for post-episiotomy pain. It has been used and tested for the treatment of herpes simplex infections as lysine seems to aid antiviral responses. One of the ways it may play a helpful role is by interfering with the cell's ability to absorb arginine. Together lysine and arginine become allies in the immune system although they function in quite different ways. In fact, they are a bit of the Yin and the Yang when it comes to immune function. For this reason, a good balance of lysine and arginine intake can be helpful for the immune system.

Fatty Acids

Dietary fatty acids come in many different forms. They are named by categories based on their chemical structures. Those called saturated fatty acids (SFAs) are generally less desirable because they can raise cholesterol in many individuals and are associated with an elevated risk of immune/inflammatory-related diseases like atherosclerosis. Transfatty acids are also bad for cholesterol levels and inflammation. In contrast, polyunsaturated fatty acids (PUFAs) as part of a balanced diet tend to be helpful against cholesterol. These come in two major varieties: omega-3 PUFAs and omega-6 PUFAs. Both varieties are needed. But many Western diets have too much of the omega-6 PUFAs compared to the omega-3 PUFAs. In general, a Mediterranean style diet has a balance that is more helpful for the immune system.

You and your baby need some fat for effective biological processes including the formation of cell membranes. But too much of the wrong type of fat is a pathway to excessive inflammation, recurrent infections, metabolic problems and other diseases. Diets are often characterized by their PUFA to SFA ratio (P:S). In general, you need to be careful not to have SFAs greatly exceed PUFAs. But even among the PUFAs, the two types have significant differences immunologically. Omega-6 fatty acids can end up producing arachidonic acid (AA), the cell surface molecule that starts the ball rolling in creating inflammation. In fact, the entire reason for taking aspirin is to reduce the products made from AA that cause fever, swelling and eventually tissue damage. And too much omega-6 PUFAs pushes the developing immune system toward Th2 responses and allergy.

In contrast, omega-3 PUFAs are protective against allergy and help the infant achieve a better immune balance. What are good sources of omega-3 PUFAs? Fish oil supplements and mother's milk. These help reduce inflammation. Additionally, they appear to reduce the risk of childhood allergy and give your child a better chance for a useful immune balance. Just be sure you steer clear of the fish contaminants like mercury, PCBs and rancid oil when getting extra fish oil.

Too Little or Too Much Food

Much of the preceding information in this chapter is based largely on how dietary components are known to affect the adult immune system. Not surprisingly, some dietary factors appear to be even more important during immune development. Too little of some dietary components or too much of others can result in childhood immune dysfunction. Maternal under-nutrition (protein and/or calories) reduces fetal growth and also negatively impacts the infant's immune system. Researchers recently described how early nutrition is capable of programming the immune system for effective balance and function or for immune dysfunction. Poor nutrition during both pregnancy and/or formula feeding of the infant raises the risk of childhood allergic disease. In contrast, breastfeeding is protective against certain autoimmune diseases and allergic diseases in certain populations of children. Therefore, attention to healthful nutrition during the pregnancy, throughout lactation and for the young child sets the stage for healthy immune performance in later life.

If undernutrition is a concern so is overeating. Excessive food consumption resulting in excessive intake of certain nutrients can cause problems for the immune system that may affect several parts of the body. One of the most common outcomes is hyper-inflammation. If your body has excess energy, it seems to get diverted into wayward inflammatory cell activity. In this case, the macrophages and neutrophils basically roam around burning the excess energy but also causing indiscriminate tissue destruction. You create your own "gang war" right in your own body. This can result in premature ageing of tissues and a higher risk of both autoimmunity and cardiovascular disease. Both too little and too much nutrient intake should be avoided when it comes to the developing immune system.

Dietary Protein

Our cells need dietary proteins to be able to get a fresh supply of amino acids, which are the building blocks of new cells. But which amino acids and in what amounts will depend upon your protein source (the type of foods you eat). For example, cow's milk has vastly different levels of the immune essential amino acids lysine and arginine compared with wheat gluten as a protein source. Your child's immune system will use both lysine and arginine. So having a varied source of dietary protein may be useful. You would not want to live only on cow's milk because your amino acid balance would be skewed and unhealthy. But the same might be true if you lived on only one type of plant with a particular predominance of some amino acids and general lack of others. Keep this in mind as you use foods as a protein source for your child's developing immune system.

Phytochemicals

Plant foodstuffs represent a major and significant dietary component. Most plants contain a variety of compounds that can affect the immune system in various ways. They fall into several different subcategories including: protein, polyphenols, isoflavones/phytoestrogens, prebiotics and, for some plants, toxic chemicals such as glycosides or oxalates. It is important to recognize that for a given age group and gender, one category of phytochemicals from a given plant source of food may he helpful for the immune system while another may cause unhelpful immune changes. For this reason it is sometimes useful to discuss the immune merits of phytochemical categories rather than whether a specific food (e.g., spinach) is necessarily good or bad. Both phytoestrogens and prebiotics are important phytochemical categories relative to the developing immune system.

Capsaicin

Capsaicin, a phenolic acid, is derived from certain plants (e.g., peppers). It is a neuroimmune modulator that has some proven medicinal properties. Research suggests it can be effective in reducing inflammation and as a topical agent in protecting against ultraviolet radiation-induced immune suppression. However, it is very potent in its effects on developing immune cells. So use should be approached with caution in the young.

Glutathione

Glutathione is in a category of plant chemicals called organosulfides. Glutathione is one of the weak links for our body when it comes to oxidative damage. It acts like an antioxidant, immune system booster and detoxifier. It helps the body repair damage from stress, poor diet, infections, medications, trauma, injury, etc. Therefore, having enough glutathione to overcome what is lost via self-damage from inflammation is important. It is produced in the body and is found in every cell, including immune cells. Found in fresh fruits, vegetables and freshly prepared meat, a balanced diet that includes these items should provide sufficient amounts. There is evidence that dietary glutathione can improve digestion in the young and reduce inflammation.

Monoterpenes

A group of phytochemicals called monoterpenes also have immunomodulatory properties. One of these chemicals, limonene, was reported to elevate several types of cell-mediated immune responses against cancer of the lymph glands in mice. It does this by helping to increase the levels of enzymes that detoxify carcinogens. It is found in citrus fruits and many other plants.

Phytic acid

Phytic acid, which is the primary storage form of phosphorus found in plants particularly in their seeds and bran, has been used in agriculture to boost the vaccine responses in young chickens. Cooking foods reduces the phytic acid content, while sprouting the grains before consumption helps it to remain intact.

Plant alkaloids

One group of chemicals of concern for the developing immune system is plant alkaloids such as caffeine and its derivative theobromine. Later in life there is some evidence suggesting that moderate caffeine intake may be useful in overcoming tumor-related immunosuppression. So caffeine intake in adults may have some benefits for immune responses. But the safety issue is far less clear for the fetal and neonatal immune system.

Quercetin

Quercetin, found largely in citrus fruits, buckwheat and onions, is among the group of plant-derived chemicals known as flavonoids. It is a definite immunomodulator. Among the effects that have been reported from the intake of quercetin are shifts in Th balance and cytokine production away from Th2 (the immature fetal state that promotes allergy) and toward Th1 (the more mature immune state that promotes cell-mediated immunity). In animals, quercetin has been reported to reduce allergic inflammation.

Resveratrol

Resveratrol is a polyphenol chemical found in red grapes. It inhibits the production of prostaglandin by acting on inflammatory cells. Scientists have shown that it inhibits systemic inflammation in neonatal animals and can act on innate immune cells to bolster cell-mediated immune responses.

Rutin

Another flavonoid, rutin, appears capable of modulating macrophage differentiation and increasing phagocytic activity. However, again there is little information concerning rutin and the developing immune system.

Phytoestrogens, Isoflavones and Soy-Based Formulas

The legume family of plants is rich in isoflavones some of which have estrogen-like properties. Genistein is an isoflavone that is also phytoestrogenic. It is found in soy and was discussed in the chapter on the Top 25 Risks. At present there is some research suggesting that significant early-life exposure to phytoestrogens, either during pregnancy or in the first few years of life, may create problems for the developing immune system. There are circumstances where soy-based formulas may be the only or a better option (as in the case of cow's milk allergy). But parents should be aware that at least some studies report adverse developmental immune effects from exposure to genistein and other phytoestrogens. This is not surprising given: 1) the sensitivity of the developing immune system to environmental modulation and 2) the presence of hormone receptors on developing immune cells. Note that there are circumstances (e.g., peri- and menopausal women) in life where the intake of phytoestrogens is often helpful. The cautionary comments here are only meant to apply to the developing immune system.

Prebiotics

Prebiotics were previously introduced in the chapter on postnatal strategies. They are a relatively new dietary aid, are complex carbohydrate molecules in foods that you do not digest but that help both the gut's natural bacteria to grow and help the developing immune system to mature. They particularly help the gut flora of newborns become established and minimize the risk of food allergies. They also appear to help the newborn's innate immune system to mature rapidly and appropriately. The latter reduces the chances of recurrent infections and inappropriate inflammation. Prebiotics are found in plants (an example being cellulose) and various foodstuffs. Naturally occurring "prebiotics" are also in breast milk. Some recent trials have suggested that supplementing with prebiotics can aid digestion and immunity in the infant.

Probiotics

In contrast to prebiotics, probiotics are the bacteria themselves as previously mentioned in Chapter 14. These can be taken as supplements or via foods rich in these bacteria such as yogurt. The most commonly used are from the genera *Lactobaccillus* and *Bifidobacterium*. These bacteria are lactic acid bacteria since they convert sugars into lactic acid. The presence of these bacteria has been shown to be important in both the local immunity of the gut as well as the immune system throughout your child's body.

Conclusions

Maternal diet during pregnancy and the diet of the infant and young child help to direct the status of your child's immune system throughout his or her life. There are several factors known to be useful in promoting a well-functioning, balanced immune system. Attention to these factors, including adequate intake of vitamin D, antioxidants and omega-3 PUFAs, can help your child's immune system to mature effectively. In contrast, when other factors are a major part of the diet, such as saturated fatty acids and omega-6 poly-unsaturated fatty acids, it is a prescription for childhood immune dysfunction and the increased risk of immune-based diseases. For effective protection of your child's immune system, attention to a healthy diet should be partnered with protection against exposure to harmful chemicals, drugs and major stressors.

Overview of Dietary Factors

- The source, type and amount of dietary factors can affect the developing immune system.
- For many dietary factors, too little can be harmful and too much can be harmful as well.
- Some dietary factors and amounts that are useful in the adult may cause immune problems during the pregnancy or in the young child.

Chapter 21 — Hygiene and Pets

Introduction

Prior chapters have described how early childhood (from birth to about two to four years of age) is a period during which the child is particularly vulnerable to infections. This is not merely coincidence. The newborn has come from a sterile environment in the womb and is thrust into an environment full of germs and chemicals. Immune maturation could only go so far inside the womb in order to prevent the mother's body from rejecting the baby. Once born, the baby's immune system needs to undergo some final immune maturation processes after birth. How quickly and successfully these steps in childhood immune maturation occur greatly determines how well the baby's immune system will be able to fight off infections. To make a comparison, think of the lungs of a preterm baby. Often the lungs aren't fully developed and have to be either protected from outside germs by placing the baby in quarantine until they're more fully developed or placing the baby on ventilation until its lungs can work fully. The immune system is similar in that it is in an immature state when the full term baby is born and must go through different internal steps to help it reach a full and balanced functional capacity.

One of the theories that has been developed over past decades about how a baby's immune system fully matures has been named the "Hygiene Hypothesis." The concept behind this theory is that allowing newborns and infants to be exposed to certain germs can help their immune system to fully develop. The idea came from studies conducted in the late 1980s concerning early life environment and the risk of asthma and allergic diseases. Researchers observed that allergies like hayfever and eczema were less common among children in large families and particularly in younger children growing up with older siblings in the household. The idea was that babies of large families are likely to have a greater exposure to infectious agents (when they had older siblings in the household) than would an only child or a firstborn. The observations were broadened to include the general environment in which the baby lived and the presence of things such as bacteria and parasites (e.g., proximity to animals).

The topic of infant hygiene is approached with some trepidation. As was already discussed, early-life infections can be serious and may affect the baby's health not only in the first year or two but also for years to come. Because the newborn's immune system is immature, the impact of infections can be serious (see Chapter 18). There are counterbalances to help protect the new baby. As was discussed in the prior chapter, breast-feeding the baby can transfer helpful antibodies from the mother that can protect the child against disease. This transfer may also help the child's immune system to mature more quickly and fully. However, given the health risks from certain infections to the newborn, parents should work with their pediatrician to guard against serious infections during the first few months.

Does this mean that maintaining a "sterile" environment is best for the child's immune system? Surprisingly, the evidence says NO. In many countries, such as the United States and Britain, we have worked long and hard to clean and sanitize our homes and daycare centers to help infants avoid germs as much as possible. But the reality is that the dendritic cells and macrophages in a baby's immune system need to encounter pieces of microbes such as bacteria in order to fully mature. This microbially-stimulated maturation helps such cells be able to promote balanced immune responses in the child. The dendritic cells and macrophages have receptors on their surfaces, among those the Toll-like receptors also called TLRs, which signal the immune system to mature further when they encounter components of bacteria. Seeing these pieces of bacteria during a time when the baby is first exposed to allergens can help protect against allergic-type immune responses (such as those involving IgE and eosinophils). It also helps dendritic cells and macrophages to be more supportive in starting antiviral and antitumor responses. So if your home is too "hygienic," your baby's immune system might actually mature more slowly and may have a tendency to develop allergic responses when allergens are encountered later.

Origins of the Hygiene-Immune Dysfunction Concept

This concept of the hygiene hypothesis, where microbes are a partner in helping the baby's immune system to mature, first grew out of the German barnyard studies that showed that the population of children raised on farms in one region of Germany had a lower incidence of allergies and asthma compared with children raised a few miles down the road in an urban setting. Since that initial study, the results have been seen in other geographic comparisons.

What the Hygiene Hypothesis Says

The Hygiene Hypothesis is based on several important ideas. First, the newborn has an immature and skewed immune system under the best of circumstances. Second, unless dendritic cells and macrophages mature further and quickly shortly after birth, they are likely to promote allergic (Th2 — immature) types of responses by T and B lymphocytes. Third, exposing the newborn's immune cells to components of bacteria does three things: 1) it helps these cells mature one step further so they can promote some Th1 functions and not default to allergic responses to harmless substances, 2) because Th1 and Th2 responses are now in better balance, defense against viral infections is improved and 3) innate immunity is under better control meaning there is less chance of collateral inflammatory damage to tissues. So if a newborn's immune system has a chance to see some microbes, then when he or she later encounters allergens, the infant is less likely to respond with harmful immune reactions. Instead, the immune system now sees allergens as something uninteresting.

Because a newborn's immune system has matured during pregnancy in a sterile environment, the adjustment to microbes is both new and critical. How the baby's immune system adjusts during the early months and years of life will influence how he or she responds to early infections, whether he or she is likely to develop allergic diseases and even if he or she will be able to handle later tumor challenges. Some examples of this follow.

In a recent study in the Children's Hospital in Munich, protection against childhood asthma was associated with pig farming, drinking unpasteurized farm milk, frequently visiting animal sheds, involvement in haying activities and working with silage. But high bacterial levels in mattress dust appeared to be unhelpful. The outside, farm-based exposures appear to help the innate immune system to mature and somehow also reduce the level of the allergy-promoting antibody, IgE, in children.

Gut Microbes

Gut microbes, also called microflora (think lactobacillus that is found in yogurt), play an important role in our ability to tolerate food allergens as well as for our general immune balance in the gut. These are also considered under the chapter covering diet because gut microbes can affect our entire immune system, not just mucosal immunity and the regulation of inflammation in the gut. Essentially, the baby is born with a clean slate for gut microbes. What had been the sterile environment of the baby's gut immediately becomes populated with a wide range and number of bacteria shortly after birth. In fact, it has been estimated that more than 500 species of bacteria populate the gastrointestinal tracts of most children. This goes way beyond the few in a yogurt culture. The types of bacteria that take up residence in your baby's gut will be determined by external environment, food source(s), chemicals and drugs that alter the immune system. Plus, different sections of your child's gut will have different species of resident bacteria that are fine-tuned to digestion in that region (e.g., small intestine vs. large intestine). It is thought that the type and number of bacteria in the newborn's gut can also impact mucosal immune maturation and in turn affect the child's specific disease risks and overall health in years to come.

Limitations of the Hygiene Hypothesis

Not everyone agrees about the importance of the Hygiene Hypothesis. Some researchers have argued that the impact of neonatal microbial exposures has been overstated. However, that may be in part because some investigators only focus on one category of environmental exposure and do not account for the entire range of environmental factors that can alter immune maturation. Where there is disagreement, it usually concerns the degree or level of importance that the Hygiene Hypothesis should be given in designing health strategies.

Today, most health scientists would agree that certain components of a newborn's immune system must continue to mature after birth, and that maturation is affected by the environment the baby encounters. Additionally, immunologists recognize that when bacterial components interact with immune cell receptors, they trigger significant changes in these cells that can impact further immune maturation and function. So how might the impact of postnatal hygiene be less than might be expected? Here are some examples that illustrate how the impact of the newborn's microbial exposure and ongoing immune maturation may be lessened because of other environmental experiences and conditions.

Prenatal/Neonatal Toxicants vs. Postnatal Microbes

The Hygiene Hypothesis is really only part of the child's immune maturation playing field. It plays into the context of the status of the newborn's immune system at birth. For example, if a pregnant woman had heavy exposure to lead or mercury and the developing fetus was exposed in the womb, the newborn's dendritic cells are already impaired in their ability to fully mature. Microbial exposure at or after birth in these children may have a much reduced impact in preventing allergic disease than in children whose mothers avoided those prenatal toxic exposures. Similarly, on the subset of farms where the pregnant mothers were exposed to pesticides, microbial exposures appear to be less beneficial to the pesticide-exposed newborn and infant.

This point is reinforced by several studies. Maternal smoking during pregnancy increases the risk of childhood respiratory allergic disease. It also has the capacity to alter the Toll-like receptor patterns of stimulation on the cell surfaces of dendritic cells and macrophages in the newborn. Maternal smoking blunts some responses and freezes maturation of these cells. Therefore, the benefits of microbial exposure in newborns are likely to be greater in babies whose mothers did not smoke vs. babies whose mothers smoked.

In summary, postnatal microbial environment is likely to modify the risk of allergic disease. However, the extent to which that modification happens is also affected by the newborns' prenatal environmental exposures.

Diet vs. Postnatal Microbes

The same prenatal and postnatal interactions seem likely to hold true in considering maternal diet and the newborn's exposure to microbes. As discussed in the prior chapter, intake of omega-3 fatty acids, amino acid balance (protein sources), antioxidants, vitamins, minerals and phytoestrogens all impact the child's developing immune system. Therefore, just as in the example for toxic chemical and drug exposures, postnatal microbial exposure is likely to have a greater impact, and probably is more useful, in those children who developed where the maternal diet was supportive of balanced immune development as opposed to those infants whose mothers had a less healthy diet during the pregnancy. However, the extent of this specific difference has not been well defined to date.

Prenatal Microbial Environment vs. Neonatal Microbial Environment

If exposing the newborn to a barnyard-type of environment can be helpful to the maturation of the immune system, the value of a prenatal farming environment on the risk of allergic disease is a little more controversial. Some studies suggest a farm environment during the pregnancy is helpful in reducing the risk of allergic disease but only if the child continues to be exposed to that environment after birth. Other studies indicate that prenatal exposure to a farming environment may not affect whether or not the child develops allergies, but it is likely to mean the child won't be allergic to those allergens the mother was exposed to while pregnant (e.g., mold and mildew in hay). As mentioned previously, whether the mother is allergic herself can change this relationship.

Genetic Background vs. Postnatal Microbes

The role of genetic background is mentioned in virtually every chapter. This is because environmental exposures alone don't determine how the immune system develops. Genetic predisposition accounts for part of development. Some children who are genetically predisposed toward Th2 immune responses (a state in which the immune system remains more like that of the fetus') may not experience the same degree and spectrum of benefits from immune maturation that is aided by exposure to microbes as would the general population of children. In these children, Th1 function may never come into full balance with Th2 regardless of their postnatal microbial exposures. It is important for parents to keep in mind that their child is unique. He or she may not necessarily experience the same changes reported for the general population for each and every environmental response.

Pets in the Home

There are lots of reasons why pets in the household may or may not be a good idea for specific families. Many of the reasons involve considerations that go beyond the benefits and costs to your child's immune system. We recognize that non-immunological considerations such as other family members who are allergic to animals, time to commit to pet care, space in which to house and care for the pet, healthcare for the pet, etc. may greatly affect the family's decision process. Therefore, the following section simply provides additional information and questions that parents may find useful when considering whether to have pets in the house.

The Role of Pets in Childhood Immunity

The immunological costs and benefits of furry pets in the household for the child appear to depend upon several factors. They are: 1) whether or not the parents or siblings are allergic to pets, 2) whether the child has already experienced wheezing or allergies and 3) the age of the child when the pets are introduced into the house.

The presence of pets early in childhood can play a constructive role for helping some children's immune systems develop.

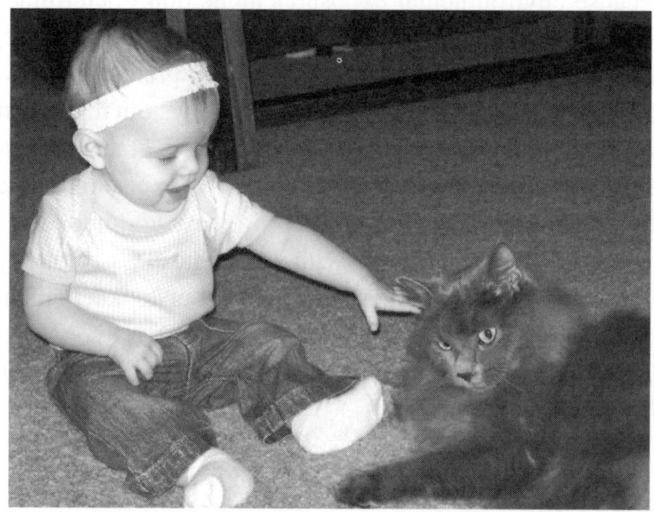

It seems that when the newborn encounters those pieces of bacteria that help the dendritic cells to mature and pet allergens are also around in the baby's environment, the child is less likely to develop pet-related allergies as he or she ages. A recent study from The Netherlands showed that infants with cats or dogs in the household were less likely to become sensitized to respiratory allergens. The presence of pets appeared to reduce the risk of allergic rhinitis (hayfever) but not necessarily the overall incidence of asthma.

However, this is not true for all children. Where both parents are allergic, this potential benefit may be non-existent due to a genetic predisposition toward being allergic. Also, if the child has already shown signs of wheezing, a possible prelude to asthma, the introduction of a pet may not be helpful.

Timing is Almost Everything

If parents are trying to decide when it might be best to have a furry pet then the general rule is as early as possible. It is far better to get the pet earlier rather than later. In fact, there appears to be a greater risk of pet related allergies when the acquisition of a furry pet is delayed until the child is six years or older than when the pet is present around the newborn/infant. So the idea of delaying the child's exposure to a furry pet (in a non-allergic household) in order to wait until the child's immune system is more mature may actually put the child at greater risk of pet-related allergies. The risk formula that has emerged is:

Newborn + Pieces of Bacteria + Pets
= More Likely Tolerance to Pet Allergens.

As before, parents should realize these results are taken from a larger population of children. Some individual children will be allergic to dogs or cats based on their genetic background and prenatal experiences. The timing of when a pet is brought into a household will not matter for these specific children who are already on a course towards allergies.

Sharing Allergies with Our Pets

Pets can also serve as sentinels of our own environment and can tell us a lot about our own health risks. While certain breeds of dogs are genetically predisposed to have allergies or autoimmune diseases (e.g., Bichon Frise dogs), the environment is also a potent factor in the immune-related diseases of our pets. They share our homes, yards, water and even occasionally our food (at least in the authors' house). Therefore, the same chemical and physical factors that may affect our immune system can influence theirs as well.

An interesting study from Germany recently described the association of a high rate of allergies in humans and a high rate of allergies in the pets that were living in the same household. Because pets share the same home environment as our children, their immune-related health issues can signal possible health risks for our children. The researchers proposed that the same environmental conditions that contribute to the risk of allergies in children also adversely affect the immune system of pets (e.g., cats, dogs, and rodents) in the household.

So the decisions parents may make to help protect their child's immune system may have the added benefit of also helping to ensure a longer and healthier life for the family's pets.

Overview of Hygiene and Pets

- Most newborns need extra Thl development and innate immune cell maturation to avoid repeated infections.
- Exposing most infants to the barnyard-type environment promotes immune maturation and protects against allergies.
- Components of bacteria aid the newborn's immune system in maturating.
- Keeping the newborn in a very sterile environment can inhibit immune maturation.
- Most infants will benefit immunologically from the presence of pets providing the parents are not allergic.
- Waiting until later in childhood to introduce pets to the household increases the risk of allergy.

Part IV — Safety Testing

Chapter 22 — Developmental Immunotoxicity Testing — Past, Present and Future

Introduction

In the event you may think the only thing not discussed in Part III of this book was the kitchen sink, no need to worry. We actually discuss our kitchen sink in the present chapter on DIT and safety testing. Many environmental factors and conditions have been identified that contribute to early life immune dysfunction and increased health risks. These were considered by category in the preceding chapters. The categories of risk factors include: 1) maternal and childhood diet, 2) prenatal, neonatal and juvenile exposure to environmental contaminants, 3) intake of certain prescription, over-the-counter (OTC) and other drugs during pregnancy (by the mom) and during childhood, 4) significant psychological stress for the pregnant mother or child (for example, bereavement, major changes in living conditions, trauma), 5) certain common infections particularly as triggers of disease and 6) exposure to certain physical factors (e.g., ultraviolet B radiation, Caesarian section delivery). The list of early-life immune risk factors is substantial and growing. In fact, a major purpose behind this book is to get the word out about those risk factors that are presently known. One of the book's goals is to provide parents, pediatricians and obstetricians with information that can assist them in making informed decisions toward the immunological well-being of their children.

The result of years of scientific testing and research by thousands of toxicologists, immunologists and epidemiologists is that we now have a "list of immune offenders." Much like Santa, we have a list of chemicals, drugs, dietary factors and conditions that we have determined are naughty or nice for immune development. But is the job of developmental immunotoxicity safety testing finished? Is the task completed except for getting the word out and helping to prevent immune-related health issues? Hardly. In fact, one could argue it has not yet even begun. The reality is that the current list of factors that are established as hazardous for the developing immune system is anything but complete and probably no more than the tip of the immune-damage iceberg. The problem is that those risk factors we presently know of cannot begin to account for the recent increases in immune-related diseases such as pediatric allergy, later life autoimmunity and inflammatory-based conditions like atherosclerosis. Because of this, we know our level of knowledge based on existing safety testing and research is inadequate. Clearly, we are missing something. We can then ask, "Are we searching enough for factors that can harm the immune system of fetuses, newborns, juveniles and adolescents?" Or alternatively ask, "Are we searching in the right way?" It appears that the answer to both of these questions is, no.

Why is this the case? Why is it proving to be so difficult to keep women who are or might become pregnant and our children out of harm's way? The answers can be found by looking at the following issues: 1) the disconnection between what is required in safety testing of drugs and chemicals and the increasing risk of immune-based diseases in children, 2) the overall goals of prior and current safety testing and 3) the nature of the testing approaches used. The rest of this chapter is a discussion of these three issues.

At the heart of issue #1 is the following disconnect or paradox:

Childhood immune-based diseases have been on the rise, but DIT safety testing is not required for the approval of drugs and chemicals (except in the case of a few pesticides and by special request). Since DIT testing is not required, it is rarely done.

The concern is that if we do not even look for those additional environmental risk factors that may be causing childhood allergic, autoimmune, inflammatory and infectious diseases, we are not likely to find them. That impairs our ability to reduce the occurrence of these diseases in our children.

Identifying Danger: The Sieve Approach

Certainly part of the answer connected to issue #2 (goals of safety testing) lies in the historic goals of required safety testing, its sieve-like features and its lingering priorities. The safety testing approach presently required (e.g., as required by regulatory agencies such as the FDA) has links to a time when overt toxicity (such as birth defects, fetal and infant death and significant reproductive damage) was the foremost concern. Environmental risk factors that produce those types of changes are among the easiest to identify and required safety testing has done an impressive job in identifying those overt risks and protecting our children from them. Additionally, once the hazards are identified they can be examined more closely. That is a success story given the goal.

In a household analogy we will use, those easily-seen overt toxic risk factors are the equivalent to the very largest stones in the bottom of a fish tank. As stones go, the largest of them are easy to see but are also less numerous than the much smaller pebbles and chips. When we clean our fish tank, the very largest stones are the least likely to be overlooked and are also the least likely to be flushed down the kitchen sink (there is the kitchen sink) and cause problems in the drain.

The question is: Is a goal or priority steeped in tradition and history the one that is most useful now in protecting our children from the current disease challenges?

Looking Beyond the Obvious

Back to our sieve analogy, if we use a standard sieve to remove the largest few stones in our fish tank during cleaning, is it then safe simply to dump all the rest of the fish tank material down the kitchen sink? Many of the rest of the stones seem so small and are almost out of sight (at least gauged by the authors' middle-aged eyesight). But we have personally conducted this experiment in our family with our very own kitchen sink.

The only good news to report is that it boosted the local economy of our plumbers. Those small pebbles passing through a sieve that was designed to catch only the very largest stones insidiously accumulated in the plumbing causing significant damage and leading to some rather expensive repairs. So what we don't see and don't catch can still hurt us.

If most required safety testing protocols are only capable of recognizing the equivalent of the very largest stones in the fish tank, that is a problem unless other approaches are used to identify those "smaller" immunotoxic hazards. Those smaller stones flowing though our sieve and into the plumbing of our house are akin to the environmental risk factors we are likely missing in currently required immune safety testing.

As is discussed in the following section, we can have a better testing system for keeping children out of harm's way. But that requires change. Some change appears to be happening, but it is ever so slow. The impetus that is needed is for parents, physicians and researchers of a like mind to come together and emphasize the benefits of seeing those smaller stones. We can and should reduce the rate of childhood immune-based disease and actually screening for developmental immunotoxicity would be a good starting point.

Safety Testing: Is It Really Relevant to Childhood Immune Health Concerns?

Since we have already discussed issues #1 and #2 and have literally hit rock bottom in the fish tank, that leaves only issue #3, "safety testing approaches," to discuss. This issue has two parts: what is tested? And how it is tested? The reality is that when immunotoxicity testing is done, it is almost always done using adults. Of course, we know that the developing immune system is significantly more sensitive than that of the adult and that unique immune events occur prenatally that are not repeated in adults. So logic would dictate that the adult is an insensitive and rather inappropriate surrogate for determining probable immune risk for a baby. Yet, that is precisely what is done. Adults are used to predict the risk for your baby. That is one of the reasons we have suggested asking about the existence of age-relevant safety data for the immune system. In many cases, the only immunotoxicity data available are from adults. That is not particularly helpful when our concern as parents or parent-to-be is for exposure of the pregnant mom or infant. So having safety testing that is actually relevant is useful. This point is further emphasized in the following box.

Major Ways We Can Miss Developmental Immunotoxicity (DIT)

- Some drugs and chemicals are never directly screened for immune effects. Are they safe for your baby's immune system?
- Other drugs and chemicals are only screened for adult immune system damage. Could they disrupt immune development?
- Safety testing often examines a resting immune system. Will that predict what will happen when your child's immune system must fight an infection?

We are down to the second part of issue #2: how is safety testing done? This question focuses on the relevance of the immune evaluation in safety testing and the likelihood it will tell us about risk of the childhood immune diseases of greatest concern. Even when developmental immunotoxicity safety testing is performed, the easiest, least expensive and quite common types of tests are those that: 1) measure changes in the way immune-related organs appear and 2) are run without incorporating something like a virus (that everyone is exposed to often) or vaccinations (that everyone experiences particularly in childhood). Mere appearance of an organ does not necessarily tell us how the immune system will function. Additionally, if the tests are run on an immune system that has never tried to fight off an illness or create antibodies in response to a vaccination, such a test system does not address the concerns for our children. We are far less concerned what an immune system looks like while it is resting, than whether it can function appropriately to protect our child against infections.

Any lack of functional testing is a serious problem because research over the past decade has shown that the organs in the immune system, such as the thymus and the spleen, can appear to be totally normal yet, when those organs and immune cells are required to actually defend against a virus, the permanent damage that has occurred to the immune system shows up as an abnormal functional response. There is currently significant debate as to what tests are needed to adequately evaluate immunotoxicity. In our opinion, the immune system needs to be challenged (e.g., with a pathogen or a vaccine) to determine if it is really functioning properly.

To emphasize the need to ask the immune system to do its job when performing DIT testing, we will use the following automotive analogy.

Car Talk and Performance-Based DIT Testing

So where does a discussion of cars come into this equation concerning developmental immune safety testing? Just as we want to avoid that lemon of a used car when car shopping, we absolutely must avoid exposing our children to environmental conditions that would subject them to a life of chronic disease. But to do that we need the most relevant safety information.

When car shopping we are concerned with the car's performance and reliability, both now and in the coming years. Our concerns over the car are no different from our concerns about early-life immune safety. Just as you want any car you buy to meet the demands of the road, with safety and reliability, the same is true for your child's immune system. You want to know that chemicals, drugs and environmental conditions your child may experience will not result in an unreliable, underperforming aka "lemon" of an immune system later in life.

As discussed, the present approach for routine immunotoxicity testing and especially for that of the developing immune system is based largely on appearance of immune-cell-containing organs. This is like buying a used car based only on how it looks while it is sitting on the dealer's lot. It may look nice and shiny from that wash and wax job they gave it, have four tires and all its bumpers (with no dents, no less) but will it function when you drive it? Who knows? Most car shoppers would agree that the appearance of a car is deceiving and does little to predict the way in which that vehicle will operate once it hits the road. Buying a car without looking under the hood, starting it, test driving it, checking its steering capabilities and, of particular interest, waiting to see if those brakes actually work when that deer leaps out in front of you would be foolhardy at best.

You want to know if it starts reliably time and time again especially in cold weather, if it handles well and has enough power to drive up those hills, provides good visibility of traffic both from the front and the side, and if it stops when needed. No less should be expected when testing chemicals and drugs for their possible adverse effects on the developing immune system.

Looks Can Deceive, Will It Run?

For this reason it becomes essential that immunotoxicity testing begin by starting the immune engine and watching the immune system perform under conditions that best simulate the certain future challenges (e.g., exposure to pathogens, allergens and stress) our children will see. Initial immunotoxicity assessment based on a structural examination of immune tissues can provide useful information. This will at least let you know that all the parts are there and that nothing is missing or has been obviously damaged. But it is far from what is needed to understand whether the immune system will actually operate as needed after being exposed to pathogens. We need to know if exposure to a chemical, drug or physical condition might impair the developing immune system for that kind of function. A useful guide for the car and the developing immune system is: don't buy a car without the test drive and don't assume a chemical, drug, dietary or physical factor is immunologically safe for the young until age-relevant immune functional safety data say it is.

Conclusions

In summary, this book has provided information on the "do's" and the "don'ts" for protecting your child's immune system. That information is based on the available safety testing information, laboratory research information and epidemiology study results that examine changing patterns of human disease. What this book cannot provide is information on any immune-damaging chemicals, drugs and physical factors that were never identified as potential hazards. Those are the drugs and chemicals that may have passed through the current safety testing sieve. Based on recent increases in immune-based childhood diseases, we know that there must be DIT risk factors out there beyond what is known. But to find them we must ask the right questions and perform the right safety tests: 1) tests that have relevance for our children and their immune system, 2) tests that measure real-life immune functions against the same kind of challenges (viruses, bacteria, tumor cells) that our children face and 3) tests that predict risk of the diseases we most fear (e.g., type 1 diabetes, autism, multiple sclerosis, schizophrenia, childhood leukemia, asthma, lupus, atherosclerosis, celiac disease). The goal should be to protect our children better now with the information that is available. But also to insist that safety data be collected that can reduce the prevalence of childhood immune-based disease.

Overview of Developmental Immunotoxicity Testing

- The developing immune system is more sensitive to insult than that of the adult.
- Currently only a small percentage of chemicals and drugs are tested for adult immunotoxicity.
- Far fewer chemicals or drugs are ever screened for developmental immunotoxicity.
- When DIT testing is done, it may not include functional testing using relevant immune challenges.
- Safety testing must be changed for us to identify all the environmental causes of childhood immune-based disease.

Appendix

Aluminum Compounds

Aluminum is the most common metal found in the earth's crust. Childhood exposure to some aluminum is likely since aluminum compounds are used in vaccine formulations and antacids. Obviously, pregnant women may also be exposed to aluminum-containing, antacid drugs.

Exposure to aluminum is both an immune concern and a broader health concern. Recent experimental studies suggest that when aluminum is ingested, it can promote a shift in gut mucosal immunity toward a Th2 bias that increases the risk of sensitization to food allergens. This is likely to increase the overall risk of food allergies.

Additional studies suggest the inflammasome (a component in some immune cells), which is responsible for promoting inflammation, is very sensitive in responding to aluminum adjuvants. This may help to explain part of the problems associated with aluminum but may also show a path toward safer solutions in the future.

Some evidence suggests that accumulation of aluminum, particularly in the brain, is associated with Alzheimer's disease. Aluminum in drinking water is another possible source of exposure. Given that Alzheimer's disease is a condition that usually occurs in later life, but is thought to involve early life risks factors, exposure to aluminum beginning in childhood would be a concern.

Asbestos

Asbestos is a fibrous mineral material that was once used for insulation and as a fire retardant. Its high melting point made it desirable as a heat-resistant building material. It is well known as an immunotoxicant and promotes lung cancer. Since the 1980s, we have known that asbestos workers exhibit severe immune alterations. By the late 1980s to early 1990s, asbestos use was significantly reduced through actions of the EPA and the courts. However, it has not been completely banned and continues to appear in some products such as brake pads and ceiling tiles. Talc and vermiculite can also contain asbestos. Additionally, exposure can still occur from the continuing presence of older insulation materials and hair dryers (the large hood type commonly used in hair salons) that contain asbestos.

Exposure to asbestos has been linked to inflammation of the lungs resulting in fibrosis and cancer. However, asbestos itself is not a mutagen. It produces lung disease through an interaction with immune cells, particularly macrophages in the lung. Once engulfed by macrophages, asbestos fibers interact with something inside the macrophage called an inflammasome. This interaction leads to the production of both proinflammatory cytokines and oxygen radicals. Over time, lung tissue gets damaged extensively and repeatedly. Attempts by immune cells to repair damage result in functional lung tissue being replaced by what is similar to scar tissue causing the lungs to lose functional capacity. As the oxygen radicals continue to be produced, they cause mutations in the DNA significantly raising the risk of lung cancer.

In effect, misregulated and "angry" macrophages that are unable to successfully digest the asbestos fibers are at the center of the lung damage and resulting cancer. This key point concerning macrophages' ability to digest inhaled fibers is also supported by other observations. Fibrous materials that are similar to asbestos but which are digested by macrophages do not produce lung fibrosis and cancer after they are inhaled. Those fibers are simply taken up by lung macrophages, digested and removed.

For children, asbestos is likely to have similar effects to those in the adult. However, it is important to recognize that the respiratory system does not completely mature until adulthood. Therefore, the outcome of exposure to respiratory toxins is often more severe in children. Asbestos produces disease based in part on the duration of chronic inflammation in the lung. This plays out over decades of life. So the earlier that asbestos is taken up by lung macrophages and that inflammation progresses, the greater the likelihood that inflammation-driven lung disease will arise in the individual.

The effects of prenatal exposure to asbestos are uncertain. However, because the adverse effects from asbestos exposure are generally focused on the lungs, it is possible that the presence of asbestos in the mother would not present additional prenatal health risks for the offspring.

Benzene

Benzene is an organic chemical in the category called aromatic hydrocarbons. It is normally found in crude oil and has been extensively used as a solvent. Benzene in various forms has been known for centuries, and it was first produced on an industrial scale beginning in the 19th century. The discovery of the chemical structure of benzene was considered a monumental advance in the field of chemistry. The compound went on to have a remarkable array of applications.

In the early to mid 20th century, benzene was among the preferred lab ware rinses used in chemistry labs. It was effective at removing traces of other chemicals from glassware. It was also used in the process for decaffeinating coffee, in after-shave lotions and in gasoline. It is still emitted in tobacco smoke. Of course, we now know that benzene is a human carcinogen. Sufficient exposure will cause leukemia.

In the body, benzene is metabolized into several different compounds some of which cause DNA mutations. Some of the compounds are also potent toxicants that 1) cause immune-related cancers (leukemias) by damaging bone marrow cells and 2) suppress immune function.

Despite a reduction in use, benzene exposure of pregnant women and children remains a concern. Benzene is still found in asphalt, charcoal lighter fluid, glues, adhesives, rubber cement, furniture refinishers, some lawn care products, automotive products, household insecticides and some inks. Additionally, exposure to benzene occurs from cigarette smoke. Parents can take several steps to reduce possible exposure to benzene. These include: 1) avoid tobacco smoke, 2) check household, lawn and automotive products for benzene and 3) check the surrounding neighborhood history for prior industrial use of benzene and environmental contamination.

Beryllium

Beryllium is a relatively light yet strong metal that occurs naturally as an element. It has properties that make it particularly useful in high-tech applications, in part, because of its electrical and thermal conductivity properties. Most exposure to beryllium occurs through the burning of fossil fuels, through food and through industrial production of consumer products. The most serious concern is occupational exposure, so the risk to children is not as great as with other metals. However, workers exposed to beryllium can bring it home to their families. Additionally, people living near plants using beryllium can be exposed to fine particles of the metal in the air.

Breathing in beryllium and having it on the skin are the most significant health concerns. Immunologically in the lungs, beryllium acts a little like the tuberculosis bacterium and nickel combined. Macrophages respond with attempts to wall off the metal (technically called a granuloma), and T cells can respond aggressively to metal complexes. Individuals can become sensitized to beryllium and can mount an allergic response that is similar to that produced by nickel. Shortness of breath, fatigue and skin rashes may occur. However, the more serious health problem is what is known as chronic beryllium disease (CBD). This can occur months to years after allergic sensitization to the metal. This is the immune system's attempt to wall off the metal. In doing so, the lung tissue becomes scarred and non-functional.

Beryllium is most commonly found in automobile electronics, computer and electronic components, welding electrodes, golf clubs, spark plugs, industrial applications involving ceramics and engines. It is also used in aircraft brakes, landing gear, the fluorescent light industry and X-ray windows for mammography. Some low level exposure to beryllium can occur through drinking water and food.

1-Bromopropane (1-BP) — Dry Cleaning Agent

1-BP (also called n-propyl-bromide) has become a popular solvent for cleaning and degreasing uses in industrial applications and for dry cleaning clothes. In fact, in the latter use it is considered a "greener," less hazardous substitute for ozone-depleting chlorofluorocarbons and chemicals of significant health concern, such as perchloroethylene. Recent studies in experimental systems conducted in Korea indicate that 1-BP significantly depresses antibody production and the cytokines needed to support T-dependent immune responses. Additionally, 1-BP depletes glutathione, a critical link in the prevention of damage to cells and tissues by oxygen radicals.

Chlordane

Chlordane is a member of the family of organochlorine pesticides. While it is no longer used in the United States, it is still produced and used outside of the U.S. Additionally, it takes a long time for chlordane to break down in the environment meaning that some exposure in the U.S. is still possible. It was used on crops and for lawn care, as well in some chlordane-containing products that were marketed specifically to kill ants and termites.

Chlordane is a potent toxin for the immune system as well as other systems. The developing immune system is particularly sensitive, and effects can differ between males and females. Research has shown that chlordane can readily damage macrophages and cause a variety of problems with immune responses. Among the health concerns from early-life exposure to chlordane is a greater susceptibility to some infections. Other effects of moderate to high chlordane exposure include: a higher risk of prostate and breast cancer, nervous system damage, gastrointestinal problems and liver damage.

In places where chlordane is still used or might be encountered due to prior use, pregnant women and children should take action to avoid exposure.

DEET (N,N,-diethyl-m-toluamide)

The active agent in insect repellants known as DEET is a substance that is chemically called N,N,-diethyl-m-toluamide. The benefit from using

DEET is in controlling mosquitoes that can carry infectious diseases like the West Nile virus. However, adverse health risks may be associated with DEET use. Alternatives now exist (e.g., oil of lemon eucalyptus), and parents may choose to consider these.

In normal use, the product should not be ingested or allowed to enter the eyes. This means that children should not apply DEET-containing agents to themselves. Additionally, in 2003 the American Academy of Pediatrics recommended that DEET-containing products not be used on infants.

DEET has been tested in some experimental models for immunotoxicity. Both changes in lymphocyte populations and suppression of antibody responses were observed at internal concentrations that more closely resembled occupational use (two weeks of exposure). However, the study was conducted simulating adult exposure. So the possible immune effects in the young at slightly lower doses are not well known. Parents may want to choose insect control for their children that avoids products with DEET.

Diazinon

Diazinon is an organophosphate insecticide that has had a wide range of applications. While its use was dramatically restricted by the EPA in 2004–2005, it can still be found in some older products. Prior to 2004, it was used extensively by gardeners. Diazinon affects the neurological system but is also an immunotoxicant. Experimental information suggests that exposure is likely to cause major shifts in cytokine production by T lymphocytes in such a way that resistance to certain infections is reduced and the risk of allergic disease is increased.

Diazepam

Diazepam (first marketed under the trade name, Valium) is a drug used to treat anxiety, seizures, muscle spasms, sleep problems, and drug withdrawal symptoms. It is technically called a benzodiazepine. Several pharmaceutical companies have marketed benzodiazepine derivatives. Drugs in this class act by enhancing the effects of gamma-aminobutyric acid (GABA), a neurotransmitter, in the brain. In humans, diazepam appears to cross the placenta, and it may be transferred to the infant during nursing.

Both prenatal and early neonatal exposure of animals to diazepam has been reported to alter immune function later in adults. Early neonatal exposure was reported to suppress both antibody production and cell-mediated immune responses. Exposure in utero was found to suppress antibody responses, cell-mediated immunity and the capacity of macrophages for phagocytosis.

Ethylene Glycol

Ethylene glycol is an alcohol-like substance that is used in antifreeze for cars, liquid-cooled computers, shoe polish and some inks and dyes (note: see the section on tattoos). It is also used in the production of plastics like soft drink bottles, though it is unlikely it would leak out during use. Much of the health concerns are for ingesting ethylene glycol. Its metabolites can produce neurotoxicity and harmful effects on the kidneys. However, it is also a potent toxicant for the developing immune system. Early life exposure to ethylene glycol causes depletion of thymocytes.

Gold

Gold is not a major exposure problem for children. However, gold salts have been used as medications for some diseases and occupational exposure occurs among goldsmiths. Additionally, some gold cake decorations are marketed as edible.

Exposure to gold salts appears to promote some forms of autoimmune disease such as autoimmune kidney disease (called autoimmune glomerulonephropathy). However, genetic background may be important in determining who is most at risk. Additionally, some evidence suggests that exposure to gold either in goldsmithing or through medications may lead to lung disease.

Lindane (Lice Treatment)

Lindane is used in medications to treat lice and scabies. For example, lindane-containing shampoos have been applied to treat infections of head lice. Though not a first course of treatment, lindane is often used as a second wave of treatment. It is a neurotoxin and affects the immune system. Children are at the highest risk for health problems following use of lindane and are the most likely to need treatment particularly for head lice. According to the FDA, seizures and death can follow exposure.

In model studies, lindane was shown to increase oxidative stress and damage by oxygen radicals within the immune system, affecting T cells as well as other cells. Results suggest that exposure can reduce both cell-mediated immunity and antibody responses.

Mancozeb

Mancozeb is a carbamate derivative compound that also includes zinc salts in some formulations. It is used extensively as a fungicide to combat fungal diseases in tomato plants, potato blight, rust spots on roses and scab on apples and pears. Studies in humans exposed through agricultural practices suggest that some Mancozeb exposures can be hazardous for the immune system. Among agricultural workers, Mancozeb suppresses the immune system's ability to make the cytokines needed for macrophages to ramp up and fight off invading bacteria.

While the human immunotoxicity results were obtained using workers exposed to somewhat higher levels of Mancozeb than would be encountered by most gardeners, the heightened sensitivity of the developing immune system also needs to be considered. The human results suggest that pregnant women and children need to take extra care to avoid being exposed to Mancozeb.

New Carpets

Old carpet removal and new carpet installation represent an underappreciated opportunity for immunotoxic exposure of the entire family. The most serious problems are also largely avoidable with some extra planning and care. Removal of old carpets during home or office renovations can enable all of the prior allergens, mold toxins and chemicals that have accumulated in the carpet over the years to be released in one major burst.

This can provide significant insults to the immune and respiratory systems as well as the skin and eyes. Old carpet removal is best treated as a type of hazardous waste operation, and the area involved should be handled as a zone that will need significant cleanup before humans can return to living in that room or area. Wearing face masks during the removal process can protect against breathing in contaminants from the old carpet. Additionally, protect the eyes by wearing safety glasses, wear clothes that cover as much skin as possible and wear gloves while handling the carpet. Also, take care to wash all clothing immediately.

Some care needs to be taken not to spread the old carpet's "chemical history" throughout portions of the house that are not involved in the actual renovation. Otherwise, the adverse health effects may continue long after the old carpet has left the property. Concern comes from a wide range of substances in old carpets. This range can include: dust mites, bacteria, pesticides and herbicides, heavy metals, synthetic airborne particles and mold toxins.

The choice of installing new carpets vs. other flooring options is a personal one, and we would not recommend for or against that choice. However, new carpet installation leads to short term exposure to several volatile organic compounds (VOCs) that can also be hazardous. It should be noted that most of the exposure to VOCs comes from the glue backing used on carpets rather than the carpet fibers themselves. Among the chemicals that can be emitted are: styrene, toluene, benzene, formaldehyde, ethyl benzene and acetone. Most of these are toxic for the immune system if exposure is high enough.

There are things you can do to minimize exposure. For example, the majority of the release of these toxic chemicals into your home or office air comes within the first 24 hours after the carpet has been installed. About 80–90% of the emissions have occurred within one week of installation. Opening windows in the room being recarpeted for the first 24 hours is a must. After that time, opening the windows daily for a week is helpful. Ideally, pregnant women and children should be kept away from the site for at least a day (while it is actively being aired out). With some planning and care, the risks of exposure to toxic chemicals associated with new carpets can be reduced.

Organotins

Organotins include several different tin-based compounds that are found in anti-fouling marine paints and are used in the production of polyvinyl chloride (PVC) tubes and bottles. The two most commonly encountered organotins are tributyltin (which has been banned because of health effects) and dibutyltin (DBT). Swiss and California researchers recently found that DBT interacts with the glucocorticoid receptor to prevent suppression of the proinflammatory cytokines IL-6 and TNF-alpha after the immune system has been exposed to a bacterium. This normally occurring reduction of the inflammation-promoting cytokines is important in bringing the inflammatory response to a halt when it is no longer needed. Since DBT blocks the ramping down of the inflammatory response, there is a concern that it might lead to inflammatory-based disease. For developmental exposures with DBT, the information is less clear. In one study, overt DIT was not found following exposure. However, proinflammatory cytokine production and/or inflammatory responses were not evaluated in that study.

Significant evidence suggests that tributyltin is an immunotoxicant in the young, and that the developing immune system is more sensitive than that of the adult. Researchers have found that early-life exposure to tributyltin causes the thymus to atrophy and suppresses both T cell responses and natural killer cell activity.

While tributyltins have been gradually phased out of marine paints (between 2003–2008), they remain a marine pollutant.

Other Organophosphate Pesticides

Other organophosphate pesticides (OP) such as parathion, chlorpyrifos, and malathion have received widespread use. These all appear to affect the immune system based on data obtained from a wide variety of species. The issue of human immunotoxicity remains somewhat controversial. However, given the diverse number of species that have exhibited OP-induced immunotoxicity and the capacity of these chemicals to promote apoptosis (programmed cell death) among human immune cells, it is safer for parents to consider these pesticides as probable immune hazards.

Minimizing exposure of pregnant women and children is a useful part of the strategy for protecting the child's immune system.

Palladium

Palladium is from the same group of metals as platinum. The data are limited regarding palladium and immune effects including the potential risk of DIT. One study among students in Germany found that those suffering from immune and thyroid diseases had high urinary levels of palladium compared with the general population. In adults, palladium and palladium-containing compounds can produce allergic sensitization, asthma and skin disorders. This suggests that exposing children to palladium is likely to follow a similar pattern of concern to that of platinum. Palladium is found in a lot of electronics: computers, cell phones, multi-layer ceramic capacitors, component plating, low voltage electrical contacts and SED/OLED/LCD televisions. It is also used in dentistry, medicine, hydrogen purification, chemical applications and groundwater treatment plants. Palladium is key in the technology for fuel cells that combines hydrogen and oxygen in producing electricity.

Phosphamidon

Phosphamidon is another organophosphate insecticide that is used in several countries in the world including the United States. It can be applied either by ground application or through spraying on vegetable, fruit and field crops. The U.S. National Toxicology Program studies suggested that phosphamidon was not a carcinogen. However, recent experimental studies in India reported that exposure to relatively low levels of the insecticide caused suppression of both cell-mediated immunity and antibody responses.

Platinum

Platinum is used in jewelry as well as in catalytic converters in automobiles. Individuals are also exposed via the refining and use of platinum salts. Platinum salts are used as antitumor drugs in the fight against cancer. Exposure to platinum has been reported to increase the risk of auto antibody production and to produce asthma and other allergic responses. Because many women may delay pregnancy and could be administered platinum salts as a therapeutic (cisplatin) while pregnant, there is concern about the potential risks involved with fetal exposure. Drugs with platinum salts like cisplatin have the ability to cause apoptosis (programmed cell death). This can slow the growth of a cancer but may also produce negative effects on proliferating cells (such as some immune cells).

Polybrominated Biphenyls (PBBs; Flame Retardants)

PBBs are flame retardant chemicals that were used in consumer products to make them harder to burn as a protection against the spread of fire. Because of their toxicity, they are no longer produced. However, they degrade very slowly in the environment, so they are still a problem based on their presence in a variety of products (e.g., computer monitors, televisions). Additionally, like PCBs, PBBs can accumulate in the food chain. Their impact on the developing immune system appears to be similar to that of PCBs. For this reason they remain a concern.

Pthalates

Pthalates are a group of chemicals added to plastics to make them more flexible. They can be found in the coating of pharmaceutical pills, shower curtains, electronics, glues and adhesives, nail polish, perfumes, pesticides and medical devices. Some PVC products also contain pthalates such as plumbing and PVC shower curtains. Diet and inhalation are the most obvious routes of exposure.

The health concern with phthalates is that they act as anti-androgens in the body. As such they block the action of testosterone. This can affect not only males but also females because a certain level of testosterone is needed in females for the production of estrogen, which is derived from testosterone in the hormone cascade.

Pthalates are both a developmental and a reproductive toxicant. Additionally, they have been implicated in the development of diabetes. Their role in immune dysfunction is unclear at present. Some studies have reported associations between pthalate exposure in children and asthma while others have seen little evidence for prenatal-neonatal immune effects. For this reason, the significance of phthalates in DIT is unclear at present. Hence, they have been listed under the "other concerns" rather than in the Top 25 Risks.

Propanil

Propanil, 3,4-dichloropropionanilide, is one of the more commonly used herbicides in the United States. It is particularly effective against broadleaf weeds in rice. Results from both experimental models and in agricultural workers suggest that exposure to propanil can alter the immune system. In research propanil was found to be a potent inhibitor of cell-mediated immunity. A research team studying agricultural workers found that propanil exposure altered both cytokine production and lymphocyte proliferation.

Pyrethroid Insecticides

The pyrethroid insecticides are a relative new class of chemicals that are man-made but similar to a chemical found in chrysanthemums. They are used to control a variety of insects but in particular, mosquitoes. Cypermethrin and deltamethrin are some of the major chemical names found among the pyrethroids. Few, if any, developmental studies have been conducted for immunotoxicity. The primary concern stems solely from adult tests. These tests, however, suggest that exposure to pyrethroids can affect the thymus and natural killer cell numbers. Additionally, some pyrethroid preparations contain potential allergens, and some individuals may have allergic reactions when exposed to them. Note, it may not be the pyrethroid chemical itself that is the problem but rather a minor contaminant in some preparations. For this reason, other synthetic pyrethroids may not have the same risk for inducing allergic reactions.

While they have not been proven to be a problem for the developing immune system, their immunomodulating activity in adults makes them worrisome. Additionally, their use is widespread. Therefore, some exposure of children is likely. Beyond mosquito control, there are other exposure opportunities. For example, pyrethroid-embedding in mattresses was suggested as a method to reduce the level of dust mites and related allergies.

Respiratory Syncytial Virus (RSV) Infection

RSV is a common virus that infects the airways. It is classified as a single-stranded RNA virus and has some similarities to the viruses that produce mumps and measles. In most people, the infection clears in one to two weeks and the airways recover to normal. However, infection in some infants and elderly can lead to complications including brochiolitis or the more serious outcome, pneumonia, in these higher risk groups. According to the United States Centers for Disease Control (CDC) most children will be infected with RSV by their second birthday. No effective vaccines currently exist for this virus. So why is RSV infection a concern relative to childhood immunological risk?

It turns out that, if the infection is severe and occurs within the first few months after birth, the child has a much higher risk of asthma and recurrent wheezing. We do not know what determines whether the infection will be severe and early in some infants. Is the severe viral infection the tipping point of environmental insults that result in childhood asthma? Or do the prior environment and genetic conditions that predispose for childhood asthma mean the infant will have a severe infection when exposed to RSV? We do not know which answer is correct.

It could be prenatal environment, postnatal influences, genetic background or all of the above. It is clear that a milder and later experience with this virus can help reduce the risk of the child developing asthma. Complete prevention of RSV is virtually impossible. But parents may be able to reduce the odds of an early infection with some attention to possible opportunities for exposure. There is some evidence that babies born in the fall are at a higher risk because they will enter the winter cold season at a younger age than babies born in the spring. By knowing this, if parents take extra precautions with a baby born in the fall, it could help them avoid an early RSV infection.

Continued breastfeeding may be helpful, but this has not been proven. The months between when the mother's transferred antibodies disappear and the baby is more immunologically mature seem to be the period of greatest risk. Therefore, a longer period of antibody transfer through breast milk could help to minimize the chance that RSV infection is early and severe in your baby.

Silica Dust

Silica is a naturally occurring substance that is found in rocks and sand. It is not the most obvious problem for children but parents should be aware of its danger for the immune system. Silica dust can found in building materials, mining operations, pottery crafting, basically anything that might involve chipping or grinding with stone or sand. A child's exposure would be more likely to occur with home renovation and construction projects or with pottery crafts. Silica dust acts similarly to asbestos. When it is breathed in, it accumulates in lung macrophages. This sets off a frustrating, prolonged inflammatory response that damages the lungs and produces a category of symptoms called "silicosis." The lungs are set up for increased susceptibility to bacterial infection, pneumonia, and even tuberculosis.

Tattoos

Parents should be aware that tattoos may contain a variety of toxins that can present problems for immune cells as well as for the skin. Historically, tattoos were applied using natural dyes like woad, a favorite of the Celts. But modern tattoos including the carriers used as solvents for the dyes can contain many of the toxins discussed in the prior chapters. Among the chemicals that are often found in tattoos are heavy metals, synthetic dyes, aldehyde and alcohol.

Most people probably do not realize why permanent tattoos last so long. It is because long-lived skin macrophages and macrophage-like cells take up the dye particles. They then sit for decades as skin decoration. Of course these are immune cells that are not being used for host defense once the "immune wallpaper" is hung. Not all tattoos are unsafe. But some certainly are a problem both from the perspective of toxicity as well as from the risk of puncture-associated infection.

There is also the element of tattoo removal should the individual no longer desire to keep their tattoos in place. Once the cells are burst and release their dye, the dye is now free to travel throughout the body and could cause potential immune system damage.

Therapeutic Proteins

Therapeutic proteins are human proteins that are engineered in the lab for pharmaceutical use and are primarily biotech drugs. They are desirable as drugs because in general, they have fewer safety concerns compared with drugs that are small molecules. They include things like monoclonal antibodies, blood proteins and enzymes. Among these are immune cytokines and receptor proteins that bind to immune cytokines. Some of these are intended to act on the immune system, but they may also have surprising and unintended problematic immune effects.

Recently, some of these proteins that were designed to correct problems with inflammation have actually caused serious, life-threatening immune complications. When administered, they caused unpredictable and massive releases of immune cytokines that led to tissue damage, organ failure and serious health outcomes. This unexpected reaction has been called a "cytokine storm." Additional complications can include a heightened risk of autoimmune reactions.

Vinyl Chloride

Vinyl chloride is produced by the breakdown of some solvents such as trichloroethylene (TCE). It can be found in liquid form, which can contaminate water or soil. It also exists as a gas. Vinyl chloride is used in the production of polyvinyl chloride (PVC), which is used in a variety of plastic products including bottles. Vinyl chloride has been found in a number of industrial waste sites and represents a significant environmental hazard. Exposure to vinyl chloride has been associated with immunotoxicity, nerve and liver damage and cancer. Most notably for the immune system, vinyl chloride appears to promote the development of an autoimmune disease called systemic sclerosis (SS). This disease is mediated, at least in part, by T lymphocytes and affects the vascular system and joints as well as internal organs including the heart, the G.I. tract, the kidneys and the lungs. It results in vascular damage and the overproduction of collagen and other proteins. Reynaud's syndrome affecting the extremities frequently occurs with SS.

Studies of immune effects following prenatal or neonatal exposure are scant. However, where age comparisons have been made on other systems, the young seem to be more sensitive to the toxic effect of vinyl chloride than are adults. Given the risk of vinyl chloride-induced autoimmunity as well as other health problems, exposure of children should be a significant concern for parents.

Glossary

Term	Definition
Acquired immunity	Immunity that is pathogen- or tumor-specific and is acquired via an infection, a vaccination or tumor growth. It is also called adaptive immunity.
Adjuvants	Substances that when included in a vaccine, enhance the acquired immune response.
Alleles	Variant forms of a gene that can be inherited. Products of different alleles can sometimes differ in activity or function.
Allergic disease	A disease resulting from immune hypersensitivity reactions against innocuous environmental antigens that pose no threat.
Anti-androgens	Substances that interfere with testosterone production, activity or signaling in the body.
Antibodies	The secreted forms of immunglobulins produced by B lymphocytes.
Antigens	Molecules that bind specifically to an antibody and also molecules that can be presented by the dendritic cells to T cells.
Apoptosis	A type of cell death that is programmed in which cells will self-degrade and not cause inflammation.
Aromatic hydrocarbons	A class of hydrocarbon that includes benzene and other chemicals that are similar to benzene.
Astrocytes	Star-shaped macrophage-like cells in the brain and neurological tissues. They support the function of nerve and brain cells.

Term	Definition
Atopy	A tendency to overproduce IgE against harmless antigens usually contributing to multiple allergic diseases.
Atrophy	Wasting away of tissues.
Autoimmune glomerulonephropathy	A form of autoimmune kidney disease.
Biomarker	Something that can be measured and which serves as an indicator of 1) the status of a tissue (healthy or diseased), 2) a biological process (e.g., an immune response) or 3) a response to therapy.
Blastocyst	A hollow structure containing clusters of cells that will form both the early embryo as well as the placenta.
Bronchiolitis	Inflammation in the bronchioles (part of the airways).
Carbamate derivative compounds	Compounds related in structure to chemicals commonly known as "urethanes." They represent a class of insecticides.
Cell-mediated immunity	An acquired immune response that is dependent upon antigen-specific T lymphocytes for host defense and not antibodies.
Central nervous system	The brain and spinal cord.
Chemotactic factors	Factors that can be detected by cells such as leukocytes and are used to guide the cells to specific locations (such as sites of infection).
Chlorinated hydrocarbons	Chemicals containing chlorine, carbon and hydrogen. They include some insecticides such as DDT as well as the dioxins (TCDD) and the polychlorinated biphenyls (PCBs).
Cytokines	Proteins made by cells that act on other cells to change their behavior. For immune cells, many cytokines are also called interleukins (meaning between leukocytes).
Cytomegalovirus	A herpes virus that infects most people. The infection is not usually a problem. But it can be life-threatening when the immune system does not function properly and infection can present an added risk during pregnancy.
Cytotoxic	An agent or process that kills cells or microbes.

Term	Definition
Defensins	Small proteins (peptides) about 35–40 amino acids long that can damage microbes by disrupting their membranes.
Developmental immunotoxicity	Toxicity of the immune system from exposure to chemical, physical or biological factors prior to adulthood (e.g., during embryonic, fetal, neonatal juvenile or adolescent development).
Developmental immunotoxicity safety testing	Testing designed to identify the hazards and characterize the risks surrounding environmental exposure of the immune system prior to adulthood.
Down-regulation	A decrease in a factor produced by cells (such as hormone receptors on a cell surface) often in response to an environmental change.
Ectoparasites	A parasite that lives outside the body such as a flea.
Effector cells	Lymphocytes that can remove pathogens from the body without needing further maturation.
Encephalopathies	Diseases or disorders of the brain.
Endocrine disrupting activity	Capacity of a factor to interfere with any part of the endocrine system.
Endocrine-disrupting chemicals	Chemicals that interfere with one or more parts of the endocrine system. This may be seen as changes in production of reproductive, thyroid, thymus or pituitary hormones.
Endogenous cannabinoids	Chemicals made by the body that use the same neurological receptors as the active compounds [e.g., tetrahydrocannabinoid (THC)] of marijuana.
Eotaxin	A substance produced by the body that attracts eosinophils to an area (usually an infection or inflammation).
Epidemiology	The science dealing with the cause, distribution and control of disease within a population.
Epidermal	Pertaining to the outermost layer of skin (known as the epidermis).
Fibrosis	Formation of fibrous-looking tissue which usually occurs during the tissue repair process subsequent to damage.

Term	Definition
Flavonoids	A group of plant chemicals that are mostly pigments containing phenols. Flavonoids can act as antioxidants.
Gamma-aminobutyric acid (GABA)	An amino acid of the central nervous system that is important in the transmission of nerve impulses. It is an inhibitory neurotransmitter that helps to induce sleep and relaxation.
Genistein	A chemical found in plants such as soy that is termed an isoflavone. It has weak estrogenic activity and is called a phytoestrogen.
Genotype	The genetic makeup of an organism. The combination of inherited alleles.
Glucocorticoid receptor	A receptor that comes in several forms and is produced by most cells of the body. It can bind cortisol and other glucocorticoids.
Glucocorticoids	Steroid hormones produced by the adrenal gland that affect both liver metabolism (predominately of sugars and proteins) as well as immune function.
Glutathione	A peptide of three amino acids that is important in protection against oxidative damage.
Glutathione peroxidase	An enzyme containing glutathione that helps to scavenge oxygen free radicals.
Gluten	A protein from wheat and other grains that is used extensively in many foods.
Glycoproteins	Molecules that contain both protein and carbohydrate (sugar).
Granulocytes	A category of leukocyte that contains granules of digestive enzymes used for killing microbes. Granulocytes include: neutrophils, basophils and eosinophils.
Granuloma	A type of localized nodule resulting from inflammation.
Hardarian gland	A gland located near the eye that is rich in B lymphocytes that secrete IgA antibodies.
Helminth parasites	A category of parasitic worms usually inhabiting the intestine that includes roundworms and tapeworms.
Hematopoietic	Pertaining to blood or blood cell formation in the body.

Term	Definition
Hepatocytes	The most common cells of the liver (often said to be parenchymal because they are the predominant cell type). These cells are important in metabolism of drugs and chemicals.
Homeostasis	Maintenance of internal stability of tissues and organs that can compensate for environmental changes to ensure stable function and health.
Host defenses	The protection of an individual against infections. They include natural barriers such as skin and mucous membranes as well as both innate and acquired immune responses.
Host resistance	Protection of humans and animals from infectious diseases and cancer.
Humoral immunity	The form of immunity that involves soluble proteins in blood and fluids. It includes antibody molecules and complement proteins.
Hyphae	Tube-like parts of the body of a fungus that is made of many cells.
Immune maturation	The progression of immune cells from infant-like stages of capacity to full function.
Immunocompetence	Capacity to produce a normal immune response when challenged.
Immunoglobulins	Proteins made by B lymphocytes that function as antibodies by binding to antigens.
Immunological memory	A unique property of the immune system to remember a prior vaccination or infection so it can respond faster and more specifically if a second exposure to the same microbe occurs.
Immunomodulating	Causing an increase or decrease in immune responses.
Immunomodulator	An agent or substance that changes (increases or decreases) immune responses.
Immunosuppressive drugs	Drugs that cause reduction in one or more types of immune function.
Immunotoxic outcomes	Problematic outcomes for the immune system as a result of environmental exposures.
Immunotoxicants	Chemicals, drugs, physical and biological agents that damage the immune system.
Infectious agents	Agents that can produce an infection such as viruses, bacteria and parasites.

Term	Definition
Inflamm-aging	Chronic, low-grade, system-wide inflammation that contributes to the aging process.
Inflammasome	A complex of proteins that is responsible for inflammatory arthritis-like conditions.
Inflammatory metabolites	Substances produced by cells after metabolism (breaking down larger molecules) that contribute to inflammation.
Innate immunity	Immune protection that is natural and does not require vaccination or exposure to an antigen. It is usually rapid but less specific than acquired immunity. Macrophages, neutrophils or natural killer cells are often involved.
Interferon-gamma	A cytokine produced by T helper 1 lymphocytes that activates macrophages.
Interleukin	A cytokine (immune hormone) that is made by white blood cells and acts on other white blood cells.
Intraepithelial lymphocytes	A specialized group of lymphocytes (mostly T cells) that protect the lining of the intestines.
Isoflavones	A family of estrogen-like chemicals found primarily in soybeans.
Keratinocytes	Cells of the living epidermis of skin and the mouth that have immune characteristics. They also produce keratin which is important to skin.
Langerhans cells	A type of dendritic (or macrophage-like) cell plentiful in the skin.
Leukocytes	White blood cells.
Lymphoid	Involving or pertaining to lymphocytes: T cells, B cells and natural killer cells.
Lysosomes	A sac inside cells that contains enzymes for digesting engulfed particles.
Lysozymes	Digestive enzymes found in the lysosomes (sacs in the cytoplasm of cells). Used to digest anything the cell internalizes.
Malabsorption	Faulty absorption of the nutrients from food by the intestines.
Maturational event	A step in a cell or organ going from an immature form to a more mature and fully functional form.

Term	Definition
Metabolism	The breaking down of substances within the body often to produce needed building blocks for life.
Metabolites	A substance that results from the metabolism process. Often a metabolite is a building block for other substances. An example is amino acids produced from the metabolism of a protein.
Metabolized	Broken down or changed as a result of metabolism.
Microbiologic flora	The naturally-occurring bacteria in a body organ or part.
Microflora	The microbes (bacteria) located in the intestine.
Microglia	A type of macrophage in the central nervous system.
Misdirected inflammation	Inflammation that causes unintended damage to normal cells, organ or tissues of the individual. This can, of itself, cause disease.
Misregulation	The inability to properly control events (in this case immune-related events) for the well-being of the individual.
Mitomycin-C	An antibiotic from the soil bacterium, *Streptomyces caespitosus,* inhibits DNA synthesis and is used in treating some infections and cancer.
Monocytes	Precursors to macrophages that are found in the blood.
Morphology	The form or structure of an organism or its parts.
Mucosal immunity	Immune protection of the mucosal areas (e.g., lining of the gut, lung, nose and mouth). It often involves IgA antibody and specialized populations of lymphocytes.
Mutagen	Agents that increase the rate of changes in DNA sequences.
Mycelium	Collection of hyphae that are usually the most visible parts of fungi.
Mycoses	Fungal infections.
Myeloid	The group of white blood cells (leukocytes) that are not lymphocytes (e.g., macrophages, basophils, eosinophils, neutrophils).

Term	Definition
Myocarditis	Inflammation of the heart muscle.
Neurochemicals	Chemicals of the nervous system.
Omentum	A sheet of fat that acts like a big bandage and hangs off the colon draping the intestines and reaching most organs of the abdomen.
Organophosphate	A chemical derivative of phosphoric and other acids. Some organophosphate compounds have been used as pesticides.
Osteoclasts	Macrophage-like cells responsible for bone resorption and remodeling.
Oxidative damage	Damage to cells and tissues caused by oxidants and various free radicals. The damage can be to cell surfaces, or to material inside cells.
Oxygen radicals	Forms of oxygen types that carry an extra electron such as the hydroxyl radical and superoxide anion.
Pathogen	An agent that causes disease. It often refers to a disease-causing bacterium, virus, fungus or parasite.
Peyer's patches	Several lymph nodes that are located in the walls of the intestines.
Phagocytosis	The process in which a cell ingests a particle and then places it in a food bubble (phagosome) inside the cell. Macrophages, dendritic cells and neutrophils are considered professional phagocytes.
Phagolysosomes	The fusion of a food vacuole or bubble (a phagosome) with a lysosome-containing bubble (lysosome) inside a cell. This is where engulfed particles are digested (basically the cell's stomach).
Phagosomes	A food vacuole (bubble) inside a cell containing a newly engulf particle.
Phytochemicals	Chemicals in plants that are considered to aid human health.
Phytoestrogen	Chemicals in plants that mimic estrogen in the body.

Term	Definition
Polyphenols	A group of antioxidant chemicals found in plants such as berries, walnuts, olives, tea leaves and grapes.
Predispose	To make susceptible to something, such as to an infection or disease.
Profession phagocytes	Cells which are best suited for and most effective at engulfing particles. They include macrophages, dendritic cells and neutrophils.
Proinflammatory cytokines	Cytokines that promote (induce or enhance) inflammation. Examples are interleukin-1, tumor necrosis factor-alpha and interleukin-6.
Prostaglandins	Hormone-like chemicals produced from a fat molecule (arachidonic acid) on the cell surfaces of macrophages and other cells. They affect inflammation, cause blood vessels and muscles to swell or shrink and affect blood pressure.
Proteolytic enzymes	Enzymes that help proteins to break down into smaller protein forms (peptides) or further to their basic building blocks (amino acids).
Protozoans	A group of single-celled organism such as amoebas.
Receptors	A chemical structure on the surface of cells or inside cells that binds to hormones, antigens, drugs, or neurotransmitters.
Roundworms	A worm that is a common gut parasite of humans.
Sick building syndrome	An illness that affects workers in office buildings. It is thought to be caused by indoor air problems and usually involves respiratory problems, skin irritation and headaches.
Surfactants	Lipid-protein substances that reduce surface tension of lung fluids and affect immune cell activity.
Synergize	To increase the activity of (e.g., another substance or cell).
Systemic sclerosis	An autoimmune disease that involves thickening of collagen-like layers around tissues (e.g., skin) and/or organs (e.g., heart, lungs).

Term	Definition
Thymus-derived lymphocytes	T cells that originate in the thymus.
Tumor necrosis factor-alpha	An inflammation promoting cytokine produced primarily by macrophages. Overproduction can cause tissue damage.
Zygote	The cell that forms after a sperm fertilizes an ovum.

Selected References and Additional Resources

Chapter 1

Gilbert SG. *A Small Dose of Toxicology: The Health Effects of Common Chemicals*. Informa Healthcare. 2004. ISBN 9780415311687, 0415311683.

Ginsberg G, Toal B. *What's Toxic, What's Not*. Berkley Trade. 2006. ISBN-13: 978-0425211946.

Lu FC, Kacew S. Lu's Basic Toxicology: Fundamentals, Target Organs, and Risk Assessment. 5th edition. Informa Healthcare. 2009.

Chapter 2

National Research Council. *Scientific Frontiers in Developmental Toxicology and Risk Assessment*. U.S. National Academy Press. Washington, DC. 2000.

World Health Organization. *International Programme on Chemical Safety. Environmental Health Criteria. Harmonized Guidance for Immunotoxicity Risk Assessment*. WHO Publications. Geneva, Switzerland. Anticipated. 2010.

Chapter 3

U.S. Centers for Disease Control and Prevention. *Epidemiology in the Classroom*. http://www.cdc.gov/excite/classroom/outbreak/answers.htm.

Chapter 4

Anthis E. Are immune system molecules brain-builders — and destroyers? *Scientific American*. March 3, 2008. http://www.scientificamerican.com/article.cfm?id=are-immune-system-molecules-build-brains.

Ferervari Z, Sakaguchi S. Peacekeepers of the immune system. *Scientific American*. October. 2006. http://www.scientificamerican.com/article.cfm?id=peacekeepers-of-the-immun.

Parham P. *The Immune System*. 3rd edition. Garland Science. London and New York. 2009.

Chapter 5

Aiba S. Dendritic cells: importance in allergy. *Allergol Int* 56: 201–208, 2007.

Holladay SD (editor). *Developmental Immunotoxicology*. CRC Press, Inc. Boca Raton, FL. 2005.

Holsapple MP, West LJ, Landreth KS. Species comparison of anatomical and functional immune system development. *Birth Defects Res B Dev Reprod Toxicol* 68(4): 321–334, 2003.

Landreth KS. Critical windows in development of the rodent immune system. *Hum Exp Toxicol* 21(9–10): 493–498, 2002.

Levy O. Innate immunity of the newborn: basic mechanisms and clinical correlates. *Nat Rev Immunol* 7(5): 379–390, 2007.

Website of the American Pregnancy Association: http://www.americanpregnancy.org/.

Website of NIH — Medline Plus — Encyclopedia — Fetal Development. http://www.nlm.nih.gov/MEDLINEPLUS/ency/article/002398.htm.

Chapter 6

Duijts L, Bakker-Jonges LE, Labout JA, Jaddoe VW, Hofman A, Steegers EA, van Dongen JJ, Hooijkaas H, Moll HA. Fetal growth influences lymphocyte subset counts at birth: the Generation R Study. *Neonatology* 95(2): 149–156, 2009.

Raghupathy R, Kalinka J. Cytokine imbalance in pregnancy complications and its modulation. *Front Biosci* 13: 985–994, 2008.

Seavey MM, Mosmann TR. Immunoregulation of fetal and anti-paternal immune responses. *Immunol Res* 40(2): 97–113, 2008.

van Mourik MS, Macklon NS, Heijnen CJ. Embryonic implantation: cytokines, adhesion molecules, and immune cells in establishing an implantation environment. *J Leukoc Biol* 85(1): 4–19, 2009.

World Health Organization. *International Programme on Chemical Safety. Environmental Health Criteria No. 237. Principles for Evaluating Health Risks in Children Associated with Exposure to Chemicals.* WHO Publications. Geneva, Switzerland. 2006.

Chapter 7

Belkaid Y, Tarbell K. Regulatory T cells in the control of host-microorganism interactions. *Annu Rev Immunol* 27: 551–589, 2009.

Burns-Naas LA, Hastings KL, Ladics GS, Makris SL, Parker GA, Holsapple MP. What's so special about the developing immune system? *Int J Toxicol* 27(2): 223–254, 2008.

Holsapple MP, West LJ, Landreth KS. Species comparison of anatomical and functional immune system development. *Birth Defects Res B Dev Reprod Toxicol* 68(4): 321–334, 2003.

Oboki K, Ohno T, Saito H, Nakae S. Th17 and allergy. *Allergol Int* 57: 121–134, 2008.

Chapter 8

Anderson LA, McMillan S, Watson RG, Monaghan, P, Gavin AT, Fox C, Murray LJ. Malignancy and mortality in a population-based cohort of patients with coeliac disease or "gluten sensitivity." *World J Gastroenterol* 13: 146–151, 2007.

Charakida M, Deanfield JE, Halcox JP. Childhood origins of arterial disease. *Curr Opin Pediatr* 19: 538–545, 2008.

Dietert RR, Etzel RA, Chen D, Halonen M, Holladay SD, Jarabek AM, Landreth K, Peden DB, Pinkerton K, Smialowicz RJ, Zoetis T. Workshop to identify critical windows of exposure for children's health: immune and respiratory systems work group summary. *Environ Health Perspect* 108(Suppl. 3): 483–490, 2000.

Dietert RR, Piepenbrink MS. Perinatal immunotoxicity: why adult exposure assessment fails to predict risk. *Environ Health Perspect* 114(4): 477–483, 2006.

Luebke RW, Chen DH, Dietert R, Yang Y, King M, Luster MI. Immunotoxicology workgroup. The comparative immunotoxicity of five selected compounds following developmental or adult exposure. *J Toxicol Environ Health B Crit Rev* 9(1): 1–26, 2006.

Luster MI, Dietert RR, Germolec DR, Luebke RW, Makris SL. Developmental immunotoxicology. In: Sonawane B, Brown R (editors). *Encyclopedia of Environmental Health*. Elsevier Ltd.: Oxford. 2009. in press.

Stix G. Is chronic inflammation the key to unlocking the mysteries of cancer? *Scientific American*. November 9, 2008. http://www.scientificamerican.com/article.cfm?id=chronic-inflammation-cancer.

Vuckovic S, Withers G, Harris M, Khalil D, Gardiner D, Flesch I, Tepes S, Greer R, Cowley D, Cotterill A, Hart DN. Decreased blood dendritic cell counts in type 1 diabetic children. *Clin Exp Immunol* 123: 281–288, 2007.

Chapter 9

Dietert RR (editor). *Immunotoxicity Testing. Methods and Protocols*. Methods in Molecular Biology series #598. Humana Press. Springer. New York. January 2010.

Luebke R, House, R, Kimber I (editors). Immunotoxicology and immunopharmacology. 3rd edition. CRC Press, Inc. Boca Raton, FL. 2007.

World Health Organization. *International Programme on Chemical Safety. Environmental Health Criteria No. 235. Dermal Absorption*. WHO Publications. Geneva, Switzerland. 2006.

Chapter 10

Dietert RR. Developmental immunotoxicology: focus on health risks. *Chem Res Toxicol* 22(1): 17–23, 2009.

Dietert RR. Developmental immunotoxicity (DIT), postnatal immune dysfunction and childhood leukemia. *Blood Cells Mol Dis* 42(2): 108–112, 2009.

Dietert RR, Dietert JM. Potential for early-life immune insult including developmental immunotoxicity in autism and autism spectrum disorders: focus on critical windows of immune vulnerability. *J Toxicol Environ Health B Crit Rev* 11(8): 660–680, 2008.

Doyle R. Asthma worldwide. *Scientific American*. June 2000.

Landrigan PJ, Forman J, Galvez M, Newman B, Engel SM, Chemtob C. Impact of September 11 World Trade Center disaster on children and pregnant women. *Mt Sinai J Med* 75: 129–134, 2008.

Libby P. Atherosclerosis: the new view. *Scientific American*. November 10, 2008. http://www.scientificamerican.com/article.cfm?id=atherosclerosis-the-new-view.

Lite J. What is Kawasaki syndrome? *Scientific American*. January 5, 2009. http://www.scientificamerican.com/article.cfm?id=what-is-kawasaki-syndrome.

Notkins AL. New predictors of disease. *Scientific American*. March 2007. http://www.scientificamerican.com/article.cfm?id=new-predictors-of-disease.

Sundel RP, Cleveland SS, Beiser AS, Newburger JW, McGill T, Baker AL, Koren G, Novak RE, Harris JP, Burns JC. Audiologic profiles of children with Kawasaki disease. *Am J Otol* 13: 512–515, 1992.

Umetsu DT, DeKruyff RH. The regulation of allergy and asthma. *Immunol Rev* 212: 238–255, 2006.

Wenner M. Autism and antibodies. *Scientific American*. June 2008. http://www.scientificamerican.com/article.cfm?id=autism-and-antibodies.

World Health Organization. *International Programme on Chemical Safety. Environmental Health Criteria No. 236. Principles and Methods for Assessing Autoimmunity Associated with Exposure to Chemicals*. WHO Publications. Geneva, Switzerland. 2006.

Yeatts K, Sly P, Shore S, Weiss S, Martinez F, Geller A, Bromberg P, Enright P, Koren H, Weissman D, Selgrade M. A brief targeted review of susceptibility factors, environmental exposures, asthma incidence, and recommendations for future asthma incidence research. *Environ Health Perspect* 114: 634–640, 2006.

Chapter 11

Arnett PA, Barwick FH, Beeney JE. Depression in multiple sclerosis: review and theoretical proposal. *J Int Neuropsychol Soc* 14: 691–724, 2008.

Burgess JA, Walters EH, Byrnes GB, Matheson MC, Jenkins MA, Wharton CL, Johns DP, Abramson MJ, Hopper JL, Dharmage SC. Childhood allergic rhinitis predicts asthma incidence and persistence to middle age: a longitudinal study. *J Allergy Clin Immunol* 120: 863–869, 2007.

Dietert RR, Zelikoff JT. Pediatric immune dysfunction and health risks following early life immune insult. *Curr Pediatr Rev* 5: 36–51, 2009.

Haller CA, Markowitz J. IBD in children: lessons for adults. *Curr Gastroenterol Rep* 9: 528–532, 2008.

Kessing LV, Harhoff M, Anderson PK. Increased rate of treatment with antidepressants in patients with multiple sclerosis. *Int Clin Psychopharmacol* 23: 54–59, 2008.

Ludvigsson JF, Ludvigsson J, Ekbom A, Montgomery SM. Celiac disease and risk of subsequent type 1 diabetes: a general population cohort study of children and adolescents. *Diabetes Care* 29: 2483–2488, 2006.

Luong A, Rolland PS. The link between allergic rhinitis and chronic otitis media with effusion in atopic patients. *Ontolarynol Clin North Am* 41: 311–323, 2008.

Potvin S, Stip E, Sepehry AA, Gendron A, Bah R, Kouassi E. Inflammatory cytokine alterations in schizophrenia: a systematic quantitative review. *Biol Psychiatry* 63: 801–808, 2008.

Ranjbaran Z, Keefer L, Stepanski E, Farhadi A, Keshavarzian A. The relevance of sleep abnormalities to chronic inflammatory conditions. *Inflamm Res* 56(2): 51–57, 2007.

Strous RD, Shoenfeld Y. To smell the immune system: olfaction, autoimmunity and brain involvement. *Autoimmun Rev* 6: 54–60, 2006.

Talan J. Depression hastens heart disease. *Scientific American*. December 2005. http://www.scientificamerican.com/article.cfm?id=depression-hastens-heart.

Warnberg J, Marcos A. Low-grade inflammation and the metabolic syndrome in children and adolescents. *Curr Opin Lipidol* 19: 11–15, 2008.

Xie J, Itzkowitz SH. Cancer in inflammatory bowel disease. *World J Gastroenterol* 14: 378–389, 2006.

Chapter 12

Herz-Piciotto I, Park HY, Dostal M, Kocan A, Trnovec T, Sram R. Prenatal exposures to persistent and non-persistent organic compounds and effects on immune system development. *Basic Clin Phamacol Toxicol* 102: 146–154, 2008.

Lemieux A, Coe CL, Carnes M. Symptom severity predicts degree of T cell activation in adult women following childhood maltreatment. *Brain Behav Res* 22: 994–1003, 2008.

Selgrade MJ. Immunotoxicity: the risk is real. *Toxicol Sci* 100(2): 328–332, 2007.

Wenner M. The danger of stress. *Scientific American*. August 15, 2008. http://www.scientificamerican.com/article.cfm?id=stress-dangers.

Weselak M, Arbickle TE, Wiglle DT, Krewski D. *In utero* pesticide exposure and childhood morbidity. *Environ Res* 103: 79–86, 2007.

Chapter 13

Alm B, Erdes L, Mollborg P, Pettersson R, Norvensius SG, Aberg N, Wennergren G. Neonatal antibiotic treatment is a risk factor for early wheezing. *Pediatrics* 121: 697–702, 2008.

Blossom SJ, Doss JC. Trichloroethylene alters central and peripheral immune function in autoimmune-prone MRL(+/+) mice following continuous developmental and early life exposure. *J Immunotoxicol* 4(2): 129–141, 2007.

DeWitt JC, Shnyra A, Badr MZ, Loveless SE, Hoban D, Frame SR, Cunard R, Anderson SE, Meade BJ, Peden-Adams MM, Luebke RW, Luster MI. Immunotoxicity of perfluorooctanoic acid and perfluorooctane sulfonate and the role of peroxisome proliferator-activated receptor alpha. *Crit Rev Toxicol* 39(1): 76–94, 2009.

Dietert RR, Lee JE, Olsen J, Fitch K, Marsh JA. Developmental immunotoxicity of dexamethasone: comparison of fetal versus adult exposures. *Toxicology* 194(1–2): 163–176, 2003.

Dietert RR, Piepenbrink MS. Lead and immune function. *Crit Rev Toxicol* 36(4): 359–385, 2006.

Fedulov AV, Leme A, Yang Z, Dahl M, Lim R, Mariani TJ, Kobzic L. Pulmonary exposure to particles during pregnancy causes increased neonatal asthma susceptibility. *Am J Respir Cell Mol Biol* 38: 57–67, 2008.

Gauthier TW, Drew-Botsch C, Falek A, Coles C, Brown LA. Maternal alcohol abuse and neonatal infection. *Alcohol Clin Exp Res* 29: 1035–1043, 2005.

Gilmour MI, Jaakkola MS, London SL, Nel AE, Rogers CA. How exposure to environmental tobacco smoke, outdoor air pollutants, and increased pollen burdens influences the incidence of asthma. *Environ Health Perspect* 114: 627–633, 2006.

Graham S. Effects of smoking may be passed down through generations. *Scientific American*. April 12, 2005. http://www.scientificamerican.com/article.cfm?id=effects-of-smoking-may-be.

Heilmann C, Grandjean P, Weihe P, Nielsen F, Budtz-Jørgensen E. Reduced antibody responses to vaccinations in children exposed to polychlorinated biphenyls. *PLoS Med* 3(8): e311, 2006. http://www.plosmedicine.org/article/info:doi/10.1371/journal.pmed.0030311.

Johansson A, Ludvigsson J, Hermansson G. Adverse health effects related to tobacco smoke exposure in a cohort of three-year olds. *Acta Paediatr* 97: 354–357, 2008.

Lovasi GS, Quinn JW, Neckerman KM, Perzanowski MS, Rundle A. Children living in areas with more street trees have lower prevalence of asthma. *J Epidemiol Commun Health* 62: 647–649, 2008.

McDonald KL, Huq SI, Lix LM, Becker AB, Kozyrskyj AL. Delay in diphtheria, pertussis, tetanus vaccination is associated with a reduced risk of childhood asthma. *J Allergy Clin Immunol* 121(3): 626–631, 2008.

Morgenstern V, Zutavern A, Cyrys J, Brockow I, Kiletzko S, Kramer U, Behrendt H, Herbarth O, von Berg A, Bauer CP, Wichmann HE, Henrich J, the GINI Study Group and the LISA Study Group. Atopic diseases, allergic sensitization, and exposure to traffic-related air pollution in children. *Am J Respir Crit Care Med* 177: 1331–1337, 2008.

Mustafa A, Holladay SD, Goff M, Witonsky SG, Kerr R, Reilly CM, Sponenberg DP, Gogal RM Jr. An enhanced postnatal autoimmune profile in 24 week-old C57BL/6 mice developmentally exposed to TCDD. *Toxicol Appl Pharmacol* 232(1): 51–59, 2008.

Ng SP, Zelikoff JT. Smoking during pregnancy: subsequent effects on offspring immune competence and disease vulnerability in later life. *Reprod Toxicol* 23: 428–437, 2007.

Ping XD, Harris FL, Brown LA, Gauthier TW. *In vivo* dysfunction of the term alveolar macrophage after *in utero* ethanol exposure. *Alcohol Clin Exp Res* 31: 308–316, 2007.

Roduit C, Scholtens S, de Jongste JC, Wijga AH, Gerritsen J, Postma DS, Brunekreef B, Hoekstra MO, Aalberse R, Smit HA. Asthma at 8 years of age in children born by Caesarean section. *Thorax* 64(2): 107–113, 2009.

Rowe AM, Brundage KM, Barnett JB. Developmental immunotoxicity of atrazine in rodents. *Basic Clin Pharmacol Toxicol* 102(2): 139–145, 2008.

Wang L, Pinkerton KE. Detrimental effects of tobacco smoke exposure during development on postnatal lung function and asthma. *Birth Defects Res C Embryo Today* 84: 54–60, 2008.

Wolnicka-Glubisz A, Noonan FP. Neonatal susceptibility to UV induced cutaneous malignant melanoma in a mouse model. *Photochem Photobiol Sci* 5(2): 254–260, 2006.

Yan H, Takamoto M, Sugane K. Exposure to Bisphenol A prenatally or in adulthood promotes T(H)2 cytokine production associated with reduction of CD4CD25 regulatory T cells. *Environ Health Perspect* 116(4): 514–519, 2008.

Chapter 14

Biello D. Children may breathe easier if antibiotics are avoided in infancy. *Scientific American*. June 12, 2007. http://www.scientificamerican.com/article.cfm?id=children-may-breathe-easier-if-antiiotics-avoided-in-infancy.

Dostert C, Pétrilli V, Van Bruggen R, Steele C, Mossman BT, Tschopp J. Innate immune activation through Nalp3 inflammasome sensing of asbestos and silica. *Science* 320(5876): 674–677, 2008.

Fowles JR, Fairbrother A, Baecher-Steppan L, Kerkvliet NI. Immunologic and endocrine effects of the flame-retardant pentabromodiphenyl ether (DE-71) in C57BL/6J mice. *Toxicology* 86(1–2): 49–61, 1994.

Graham S. Ozone linked to hardening arteries. *Scientific American*. November 7, 2003. http://www.scientificamerican.com/article.cfm?id=ozone-linked-to-hardening.

Kushima K, Oda K, Sakuma S, Furusawa S, Fujiwara M. Effect of prenatal administration of NSAIDs on the immune response in juvenile and adult rats. *Toxicology* 232(3): 257–267, 2007.

Smialowicz RJ. The rat as a model in developmental immunotoxicology. *Human Exp Toxicol* 21(9–10): 513–519, 2002.

Veraldi A, Costantini AS, Bolejack V, Miligi L, Vineis P, van Loveren H. Immunotoxic effects of chemicals: a matrix for occupational and environmental epidemiological studies. *Am J Ind Med* 49(12): 1046–1055, 2006.

Chapter 15

Dietert RR. Distinguishing environmental causes of immune dysfunction from pediatric triggers of disease. *Open Pediatr Med J* 3: 38–44, 2009. http://www.bentham.org/open/topedj/openaccess2.htm.

Greaves M. Infection, immune responses and the aetiology of childhood leukaemia. *Nat Rev Cancer* 6: 193–203, 2006.

Hansbro NG, Horvat JC, Wark PA, Hansbro PM. Understanding the mechanisms of viral induced asthma: new therapeutic directions. *Phamacol Ther* 117: 313–353, 2008.

Hogaboam JP, Moore AJ, Lawrence BP. The aryl hydrocarbon receptor affects distinct tissue compartments during ontogeny of the immune system. *Toxicol Sci* 102(1): 160–170, 2008.

Su BY, Su CY, Yu SF, Chen CJ. Incidental discovery of high systemic lupus erythematosus disease activity associated with cytomegalovirus viral activity. *Med Microbiol Immunol* 196: 165–170, 2007.

Tourdot S, Mathie S, Hussell T, *et al.* Respiratory syncytial virus infection provokes airway remodeling in allergen-exposed mice in absence of prior allergen sensitization. *Clin Exp Allergy* 38: 1016–1024, 2008.

Chapter 16

McDonald KL, Huq SI, Lix LM, Becker AB, Kozyrskyj AL. Delay in diphtheria, pertussis, tetanus vaccination is associated with a reduced risk of childhood asthma. *J Allergy Clin Immunol* 121(3): 626–631, 2008.

Chapter 17

Dietert RR, Dietert JM. Immunotoxicology and foods. In: Watson RR, Zibadi S, Victor R, Preedy VR (editors). *Dietary Components and Immune Function. Prevention and Treatment of Disease and Cancer.* Humana Press. Springer Science + Business Media LLC. New York, NY. 2009. in press.

Langley-Evans SC, Carrington LJ. Diet and the developing immune system. *Lupus* 15: 746–752, 2006.

Moeller R. Soy-based infant formulas may hinder immune system. *Scientific American.* May 21, 2002. http://www.scientificamerican.com/article.cfm?id=soy-based-infant-formulas.

Prescott SL, Dunstan JA. Prenatal fatty acid status and immune development: the pathways and the evidence. *Lipids* 42: 801–810, 2007.

Scheff J. Fact or fiction: antioxidant supplements will help you live longer. *Scientific American*. June 6, 2008. http://www.scientificamerican.com/article.cfm?id=antioxidant-supplements-will-help-you-live-longer.

Shepard D. Immunomodulation by nutraceuticals and functional foods. In: Luebke R, House R, Kimber I (editors). *Immunotoxicology and Immunopharmacology*. CRC Press, Inc. Boca Raton, FL, pp. 185–206, 2007.

Swaminithan N. When the levee breaks: protein overwhelmed by overeating leads to metabolic diseases. *Scientific American*. May 3, 2007. http://www.scientificamerican.com/article.cfm?id=protein-stops-inflammation-metabolic-diseases.

Tavera-Mendoza LE, White JH. Cell defenses and the sunshine vitamin. *Scientific American*. November 2007. http://www.scientificamerican.com/article.cfm?id=cell-defenses-and-the-sunshine-vitamin.

Chapter 18

Dietert RR, Dietert JM. Early-life immune insult and developmental immunotoxicity (DIT)-associated diseases: potential of herbal- and fungal-derived medicinals. *Curr Med Chem* 14(10): 1075–1085, 2007.

Niemi B-J. Placebo effect: a cure in the mind. *Scientific American*. February 2009. http://www.scientificamerican.com/article.cfm?id=placebo-effect-a-cure-in-the-mind.

Chapter 19

Cone M. New study: autism linked to environment. *Scientific American*. January 9, 2009. http://www.scientificamerican.com/article.cfm?id=autism-rise-driven-by-environment.

Dietert RR, Piepenbrink MS. The managed immune system: protecting the womb to delay the tomb. *Hum Exp Toxicol* 27(2): 129–134, 2008.

Dietert RR, Zelikoff JT. Early-life environment, developmental immunotoxicology, and the risk of pediatric allergic disease including asthma. *Birth Defects Res B Dev Reprod Toxicol* 83(6): 547–560, 2008.

Selgrade MK, Lemanske RF Jr, Gilmour MI, Neas LM, Ward MD, Henneberger PK, Weissman DN, Hoppin JA, Dietert RR, Sly PD, Geller AM, Enright PL,

Backus GS, Bromberg PA, Germolec DR, Yeatts KB. Induction of asthma and the environment: what we know and need to know. *Environ Health Perspect* 114(4): 615–619, 2006.

Tollanes MC, Moster D, Daltveir AK, Irgens LM. Cesarean section and risk of severe childhood asthma: a population-based cohort study. *J Pediatr* 153: 112–116, 2008.

Wenner M. Infected with insanity: could microbes cause mental illness? *Scientific American*. April 2008. http://www.scientificamerican.com/article.cfm?id=infected-with-insanity.

Chapter 20

Cooke A. Infection and autoimmunity. *Blood Cells Mol Dis* 42(2): 105–107, 2009.

Dietert RR. Distinguishing environmental causes of immune dysfunction from pediatric triggers of disease. *Open Pediatr Med J* 3: 41–47, 2009. http://www.bentham.org/open/topedj/openaccess2.htm.

Hosea Blewett HJ, Cicalo MC, Holland CD, Field CJ. The immunological components of human milk. *Adv Food Nutr Res* 54: 45–80, 2008.

Lite J. On the kid's menu: food allergies. *Scientific American*. October 22, 2008. http://www.scientificamerican.com/blog/60-second-science/post.cfm?id=on-the-kids-menu-food-allergies-2008–10–22.

Prescott SL, Smith P, Tang M, Palmer DJ, Sinn J, Huntley SJ, Cormack B, Heine RG, Gibson RA, Makrides M. The importance of early complementary feeding in the development of oral tolerance: concerns and controversies. *Pediatr Allergy Immunol* 19(5): 375–380, 2008.

Chapter 21

Adler A, Tager I, Quintero DR. Decreased prevalence of asthma among farm-reared children compared with those who are rural but not farm-reared. *J Allergy Clin Immunol* 115: 67–73, 2005.

Duramad P, Harley K, Lipsett M, Bradman A, Eskenazi B, Holland NT, Tager IB. Early environmental exposures and intracellular Th1/Th2 cytokine profiles in 24-month-old children living in an agricultural area. *Environ Health Perspect* 114: 1916–1922, 2006.

Klement E, Lysy J, Hoshen M, Avitan M, Goldin E, Israeli E. Childhood hygiene is associated with the risk for inflammatory bowel disease: a population-based study. *Am J Gastroenterol* 103: 1775–1782, 2008.

Renz H, Blumer N, Virna S, Sel S, Garn H. The immunological basis of the hygiene hypothesis. *Chem Immunol Allergy* 91: 30–48, 2006.

Somberg TC, Arora RR. Depression and heart disease: therapeutic implications. *Cardiology* 111: 75–81, 2008.

Wong K. Early exposure to pets may keep allergies away. *Scientific American.* August 28, 2002. http://www.scientificamerican.com/article.cfm?id=early-exposure-to-pets-ma.

Chapter 22

Dietert RR (editor). *Immunotoxicity Testing. Methods and Protocols.* Methods in Molecular Biology series #598. Humana Press. Springer. New York. January 2010.

Dietert RR. Developmental immunotoxicology: focus on health risks. *Chem Res Toxicol* 22(1): 17–23, 2009.

Dietert RR. Developmental immunotoxicity (DIT) in drug safety testing: matching DIT testing to adverse outcomes and childhood disease risk. *Curr Drug Saf* 3(3): 216–226, 2008.

Dietert RR. Developmental immunotoxicity testing and protection of children's health. *PLoS Med* 3(8): e296, 2006. http://www.plosmedicine.org/article/info:doi/10.1371/journal.pmed.0030296.

Herzyk DJ, Bussier JL (editors). *Immunotoxicology Strategies for Pharmaceutical Assessment.* John Wiley & Sons. Hoboken, NJ. 2008.

U.S. FDA. *Guidance for Industry: ICH S8 Immunotoxicity Studies for Human Pharmaceuticals.* Center for Drug Evaluation and Research. Rockville, MD. 2006. http://www.fda.gov/cder/guidance/6748fnl.htm.

U.S. FDA. *Guidance for Industry: Nonclinical Safety Evaluation of Pediatric Drug Products.* Center for Drug Evaluation and Research. Rockville, MD. 2006. http://www.fda.gov/cder/guidance/5671fnl.htm.

Index